WTF am I supposed to eat?

a dieter's manifesto

by C.J. English

The following content has not been rated but does contain graphic language, mature subject matter, some nudity, sexuality and irreverent, dry, sarcastic, WTF humor. If you're easily offended or have a tendency toward sending hate mail, consider reading a different book.

WTF am I supposed to eat? is the opinion of one person, not true and tested scientific facts. This is not a textbook. It's a manifesto written by someone who generally knows what she's talking about but readily admits that, in fact, she may actually know nothing. The content that follows is based on experiments she's done on herself and others. So for fuck's sake, try not to take anything too seriously.

Editor and Interior Design: Hannah Hutton Clark and Laura Bania

www.writeawaypublishing.com

Cover Design: MSPIRE

www.mspire.com

Cover Photo: Two Hearts Photography

www.twoheartsphotos.com

www.facebook.com/twoheartsphoto

Hair and Makeup: Molly Grundysen

www.facebook.com/mollygrundysen

Cover photo on location at The Aspens at Timber Creek, Fargo, ND. Courtesy of Heritage Homes.

www.heritagefargo.com

Paperback ISBN: 978-0-9863042-2-4

Digital ISBN: 978-0-9863042-3-1

Contents

To everyone who shares my dream of eating whatever you want and not getting fat, this one is for you.

Introduction

"FORGET WHAT YOU THINK YOU KNOW,

YOU MIGHT KNOW NOTHING."

Coconut or hemp milk? Wait... I haven't even tried soy milk or almond milk.

Paleo or are we still doing Atkins?

Raw nuts or roasted?

Splenda or Truvia? Or is it stevia or agave? And WTF is turbinado sugar?

What about those protein shake places, are they good for me?

Should I be eating chia seeds?

Is flax still a thing?

Steel-cut or old-fashioned oats?

What's with all these pastas?

I should be eating Greek yogurt, right?

Is red meat actually that bad for me? What if I only eat grass-fed beef? Or bison? Or venison?

You confused?

You and everyone else. You deserve to know what it really takes to lose weight, what it really takes to keep weight off, and the truth about what's actually healthy and what will fucking kill you. You also deserve to have someone relentlessly encourage you along your journey as you pursue lifelong health, preferably someone with no ties to the food industry, supplement companies or any other entity trying to make money off getting you to buy their shit. That's me. I'm a nobody with no ties, who's spent a lifetime sifting through the sea of weight-loss information and misinformation all tangled up in knots.

It has been my mission to unravel the mess and search for WTF is the truth and WTF is total bullshit. The question I've sought the answer to is this: *how can I eat whatever I want and still stay skinny... forever? I also want to look younger than I am, have as much energy as I can possibly have, and live a long, disease-free life.*

10

This lifelong quest for skinnydom has turned me into a chronic dieter, information sponge, health food nut, wine drinker, juice maker, smoothie connoisseur, but above all, a plant eater—a *mostly* plant eater.

My triumphs and pitfalls attempting to lose weight have taught me how to get and stay skinny with as little effort as possible. On the pages that follow are the things I have learned along the way.

This is my manifesto.

A public declaration of what I think I know. But through all of my experiments on myself and others, and a little bit of reading too, all I've really discovered is that I know nothing. So this book is not a scientific proclamation of facts, although I will present some to you throughout—I will also scatter a few pieces of bullshit here and there to see if you're still paying attention.

I am not a dietitian, nutritionist or food scientist. Nor do I have a renowned degree in anything you'd likely be impressed with. But I am smart. I have been *edu-mac-ated* by many a college and might even have received a few pedigrees. But mostly, I just have a kinky fetish for solving problems by thinking outside the box. Not *math* problems—I fucking hate math problems. I mean I like to figure shit out; I like to play chess and not just on a chessboard. More importantly, I have the gumption to think critically and the courage to share my observations. Without questioning what we think to be true, we will never find the real truth at all.

So here is what I *do* know... for sure.

When I'm skinny, I'm happy; when I'm fat, I'm not.

I like being skinny; even more, I like *feeling* skinny.

I hate feeling fat; I *despise* feeling fat.

Feeling fat feels like shit; being fat feels even more like shit.

Don't assume I'm as shallow as a shot glass and expect everyone to be skinny in order to be happy, quite the contrary is true. All I'm saying is that *I* prefer to feel skinny as opposed to *feeling* fat, and the only way for me to feel skinny is to actually *be* skinny. I've been both skinny and fat—my preference is clear.

So am I skinny?

Yes.

A tad muscular?

A tad.

A smidge flabby when I jump up and down naked in front of the mirror?

A smidge.

Am I fucking ripped? Jacked? Sliced?

Um... no.

If the physique you desire is the shredded look of the men and women on the cover of muscle magazines, you are reading the wrong book. No one who has the bad food behaviors that I have and is not willing to give them up could be that fit. But that is one of my secrets to how I stay skinny.

I *have* to be bad to stay skinny.

OK, the truth is that I have zero willpower—that's why I have to be bad. However, I've figured out how to work with this pesky willpower weakness. And it's not by going to the gym.

Overuse injuries and a strong aversion to going to the gym have forced me to figure out what food lifestyle works for me instead of forcing myself to exercise when it's actually quite boring. This journey has been a bitch at times; I'm not naturally skinny with a high metabolism, and I'm not blessed with bikini body genes. I have been way too fat, way too skinny, extremely unhealthy and un-sustainably overly healthy many times over. Simply put—I've been a hot mess and a not-so-hot mess. Being all over the spectrum of wellness and weight loss has been beneficial in pointing me toward balance.

Life is messy sometimes—chaotic, and crammed with too many things and never enough time. OK, it's that way all the time. But still, I have figured out that if I want to stay skinny with three kids, three friends, a full-time job, one Goldendoodle and keep an amazing marriage to an insanely hot husband (which I wrote about in the Amazon Kindle #1 Best Selling Book in Diaries and Journals, *AFFAIRYTALE, a Memoir*) weight loss has become more of an art than a science. Although science is the foundation on which sound knowledge is built, sometimes art is necessary to be able to see how things fit together. I am going to show you how I've pieced it all together, and I'll share how others have done it too. My hope is that you are able to figure out for yourself what will work and gain the clarity to know what won't.

You will not be reading about how much protein you should eat or getting recommendations on grams of carbs or calories, nor will I be citing a thousand peer reviewed studies that plants are a better food choice than animals—even though they are and I want to—I won't. Because there are a thousand other studies that say the opposite is true.

Both sides will be convincing; both sides will have facts and supporting evidence that seems overwhelmingly in their favor; and both sides will have flaws, mistakes, oversights and quite possibly will be contaminated with corruption and greed. None of that matters anyway. We aren't creatures who wholeheartedly believe in evidence. We live our lives by faith, hunches, gut feelings, opinions, and personal convictions regardless of the truth.

I won't be cramming chicken, tuna, or brown rice down your throat or telling you to exercise more. I'm not saying exercise is bad—that would be fucking stupid. However, the current approach to working out for weight loss is not working; two thirds of Americans are still overweight, one third of them obese. More on not exercising for weight loss in chapter three. Until then, if you are currently using exercise to lose weight and it's not working, cut it the fuck out. Go spend your time at the farmer's market and then in the kitchen where it'll actually pay off. You have my permission to not exercise until you are done reading this book and have reconsidered your plan.

Forget what you think you know; you might know nothing. All I know is that I actually know nothing, and when I can admit that to myself, only then do I begin to learn. So open your mind, ask yourself if what you've done or have been doing is really working or if you might have to re-think your plan.

Now...

If I skip right to telling you *what* to eat, you won't be successful at losing weight. Even when you know *what* to eat (which I'm certain most of you do) perhaps you haven't been able to stick with it.

To lose weight, I believe we have to have a meaningful understanding of *why* we should be doing something or why we should not. Meaningful is different for everybody, but eventually, something will click, hit home, rattle you to the core, and you'll realize that if you don't do what it is you need to, you and the people you love will suffer. If you don't change the way you think, it won't matter if you know *what* to eat because you won't have the internal motivation or tools to eat that way anyway. So before we discuss if almond milk is better than soy milk or whether or not you should be eating coconut oil by the spoonful, let's delve into a few tricks that may blow your mind and build the foundation for lasting weight-loss results.

As we go, I expect you to be curious, look shit up, ask questions, and don't take what I or anyone else says to be true without thinking critically and investigating for yourself. Form your own opinions—just don't form your own facts. Set free your inquisitiveness and have rigor in finding out what works for you... that is the key.

Did you catch that? That was important.

The key to weight loss is figuring out what works for *you*.

Part I:
How

Chapter 1

"THE BEST WEIGHT-LOSS PLAN WILL FIT YOU LIKE A RED CARPET DRESS—TAPED, PINNED AND HEMMED TO FIT YOUR EVERY CURVE, BULDGE, AND IMPERFECTION."

You have to create your own program.

Weight loss happens when you stop going on other people's "programs" and create your own instead. Once you have a designed a personalized weight-loss strategy, one that is integrated into your every cell—a diet you cannot go off of because it's not really a diet at all—only then, will you be successful.

Here's how to do it.

First, stop trying and re-trying the same old diets that haven't worked for you in the past. Get over it and don't even try to tell yourself *this time it'll work if I just stick with it.* Of course it will work if you stick with it—most diets do work for weight loss if you stick with it—but that's the problem: you don't stick with it.

Why? Because you haven't been honest with yourself about what you realistically can and can't do or what you are and aren't willing to give up. Did you really think you could go 30 days without eating out and working out every day at 6 a.m.? Did you really think you'd go three weeks on less carbs than a corn cob without the kernels? No—you were on someone else's program and not one that took into account your unique, sometimes weird, preferences. Anything that does not consider the things you love most or the foods you won't give up, will fail. Since no one knows you better than you, you'll have to create a plan for yourself. Once you do, your diet will not only work for you, but it will become you: it *is* you. The healthier, thinner version of you.

I will often hear this, "What do you eat? I'll just do that."

Within this question lies a widespread damaging misconception about losing weight. It implies that if so-and-so does such-and-such and you do the same, you'll both get the same results. This is what most weight-loss programs assume and understandably so. How could a diet book or program that needs to be scaled for the masses cover thousands of specific scenarios for weight loss, one for each unique reader? It can't. The information we get about what is healthy and what will help us lose weight are often over-generalized statements that assume everyone is the same and loses weight the same. We don't.

Sure, we're the same in some ways. We also have a similar biology to rats, mice, rabbits, primates, and all the other poor creatures that are forced to be our stand-ins for testing things that might be unsafe for humans. Like mascara and... weight-loss pills. *

So, does a weight-loss pill that causes fat loss in a mouse cause fat loss in a human—is that a fair comparison? What animal do you want standing in for you? My answer is none—not even another human. I don't want to be let down by trying another thingamajig that seems to work for everyone else but just doesn't work for me.

Although there are elements in common weight-loss programs that work for many people, the most successful long term weight-loss programs are not designed as one-size-fits-all. The best weight-loss plan will fit you like a red carpet dress—taped, pinned, and hemmed to fit your every curve, bulge, and imperfection; a dress that cannot be worn by anyone else because it has

---

* *We could do away with the barbaric practice of testing on animals, don't cha think?*

been sewn on you by the designer herself. The hard part is finding such a skilled designer to craft a perfectly unique dress. So if you don't have a Vera Wang of weight loss available to help you, you're going to have to figure out how to become the best damn dressmaker on your own.

A weight-loss plan that is specific to you, designed for your unique tastes, available time, preferences, and social life situations is the one that will work permanently.

This, my friends, is what we are going to attempt to do together over the course of this book—so that you never go on, or off, a *diet* ever again.

...

You'll have to get choosy.

You can't change everything. Change only what you need to in order for you to be successful, fuck the rest—for now. Changing more than you can handle at once will slow you down or prevent success altogether. But *do* be honest with yourself about this. Small changes will produce small results over a long period of time. Like your 401K. It's worth a few nickels right now, but if you're not shortsighted and let it sit for a couple decades, maybe you'll be able to buy a yacht. Or a fishing boat. Or maybe just a beach chair and some Coronas—whatever. Depends on how much you save, right? How hard you work? How much you commit to the long term goal you know will pay off big? But if you just put in a little more effort, it could mean the difference between a body that is a retirement rust bucket that creaks and can't even sit on your floor or a luxury liner who is supple, lean, and loving life till the end.

If you're on the brink of meeting the man in the sky, then by golly, you'll need to kick it in the ass and make some serious changes. But if you have some weight to lose and are not about to float through the tunnel of white light anytime soon, then prioritizing will suffice.

Weight loss is not only about knowing *what* to eat, it's about knowing yourself well. Pre-designed diet programs set you up for failure because they do not take into account unique you.

You have to be able to do what you like (most of the time) in order to be permanently successful. So... you'll have to build naughtiness into your plan. And if you do it wisely, in the right amounts, you'll lose weight while getting to eat whatever you want. *That's* when it won't seem like a diet at all.

Ideally we'd meet in person. I would ask you questions and help you come to conclusions about the reality of your willpower or lack of it, but since we most likely can't unless you move to Fargo, my goal is to preempt some of your questions. From there you'll have to decide if "this," whatever it is, will work for *you*.

In some instances, just because I've said it will work, or has worked for someone else, doesn't mean it will work for you. You'll have to do some critical thinking and discover what works in part by trial and error.

At the end of this book, someone is going to say, "Holy shit, Mary Jane, you've lost so much weight. What did you do?" The answer is simple. "I stopped going on and off diets, created my own routine, and have learned what works and what doesn't work for me. I love what I eat, and I work out when I want to."

If someone was asking me how I stay skinny, I would preface it with, "This might not work for you because it's made for my weird tastes. But I drink green tea every morning and wine every evening. Sometimes I eat nachos with jalapeños at midnight after I'm drunk, and once or twice, I've eaten so much cheese I can't shit for three days. But not often. Occasionally I've smuggled a donut, or two, into my car and ate them in secret by the railroad tracks on the outskirts of town. I've been known to hoard the left over Chinese food, and I have absolutely no willpower whatsoever against pretty much everything. But, when I'm not doing any of that, I eat really healthy. I eat plants. My diet is made up of 95 percent plants. I juice, I walk, I plan ahead when I can, and I use affirmations such as 'I like being skinny more than I like eating cheese' to remind myself to stay on track from the temptations abound. I avoid situations where I know I'll cave in and sabotage myself. I weigh myself for a slap on the ass a few times a week, and I give myself ten pounds of wiggle room before I freak out, call in sick, and then go to the gym all day."

So how the fuck is it possible for me to still be skinny doing nothing but walking and some light girly exercises on the floor?

I don't do *all* of that bad shit *all* of the time.

I do *some* of that bad shit *some* of the time.

Except wine—I do that all of the time.

The key for me is that I eat plants—it's what keeps me skinny. Lots and lots of plants. Not *only* plants, but *mostly* plants. This works for me, and I'm pretty sure this is one of those things that can work for you too. Or maybe not, because you'll have to figure that out on your own remember? But I'd recommend you give a plant-based diet a try if you want to lose weight and be optimally healthy.

There's no debate that plant eaters generally live longer, have lower weights, and suffer less major health issues. I will sprinkle my plant-eating propaganda throughout, however, I'm not going to tell you to give up anything. Well... maybe some things. But you'll have to be smart about deciding what you can and can't give up so that you're successful forever.

Since I know myself well and freely admit that I have little willpower, part of my successful skinny lifestyle is avoiding all the sabotaging food situations that I can but knowing I can't avoid them all. I am extra good when I have control over my food environment because I know there will be times when I don't. I would rather indulge my bad habits outside of my house where I have less will and more temptations than in my house where I can control what's in the fridge and pantry.

It does help that I give myself ten pounds of jiggle room to play with. Consider doing the same. I have two weights, my *on-season* weight of 115 pounds and my *off-season* weight of 125 pounds. Both are perfectly healthy weights for me. As long as I am somewhere in that range, I'm good with that.

Depending on the time of year and if I get the opportunity to wear a bikini in Hawaii or hiking gear in Alaska, I gain or lose by becoming more or less disciplined as needed. Mostly I'm less disciplined, because I fail if I try to maintain my on-season weight for too many months out of the year. This way I can screw off for most of the year and eat sweet potato fries dipped in sweet Thai chili sauce from my favorite German beer joint; then I have intermittent months of cracking down where I avoid hefeweizen, lederhosen, and hammerschlagen.

Get out your journal. Write this down. Ask yourself *"what are my three biggest weaknesses?"* The top three things that are holding you back from losing weight. This is where you will start focusing your efforts. Stop dickin' around with everything else, hit 'em where it hurts—it's time to get efficient.

Chapter 2

"FIGURE OUT WHAT YOUR BIGGEST OBSTACLE TO WEIGHT LOSS IS AND START THERE. DON'T WASTE YOUR TIME ANYWHERE ELSE."

If you were an Olympic swimmer, would your workouts consist of roller skating and frolfing? Of course not. So why waste time with anything that is not going to get you to your goal the quickest? I've excused you from exercise for the time being because it might not be the smartest place to spend your energy—right now, at least. Have you considered that maybe exercise just makes you more fucking hungry? And that if you're always hungry and don't know what to eat or lack the willpower to eat healthy anyway, you'll gain more weight than if you weren't working out?

Dr. Andrew Weil, founder and director of The Arizona Center for Integrative Medicine, wrote in his October, 2012 *Huffington Post* article, "Carbohydrate Density: A Better Guide to Weight Loss," that, "Excess exercise tends to be counterbalanced by excess hunger, exemplified by the phrase 'working up an appetite.' A few people with extraordinary willpower can resist such hunger day after day, but for the vast majority, weight loss through exercise is a flawed option."

Figure out who your number one enemy is and attack there first. Don't light up the wrong neighbor's doorstep with a flaming bag of poop if you're not 100 percent sure it's their dog who's leaving shit bombs in your yard. Figure out what your biggest obstacle to weight loss is and start there. Write it down. Don't waste your time anywhere else. We'll tackle the less important problems later when you've lost your first twenty pounds.

When clients ask, "What can I put in my morning coffee so I can still lose weight?" I say, "Do you think your morning coffee is one of the top three reasons you're not losing weight?" Usually the answer is no, and they can list three much bigger weight-loss saboteurs than coffee and cream. Which puts into perspective how insignificant their morning coffee is in comparison to their addiction to let's say... candy corn, alfredo pasta, and eating out.

Let's say Tamera has a sweet tooth not only for her morning coffee but everywhere else too, and in general when she eats, her portions could feed all of Mongolia. It would be a better use of Tamera's time, energy and resources, working on how to get *those* bad habits under control rather than focusing on a few extra calories in her morning coffee that are infinitesimal in comparison.

Now, for Roxanne, no amount of going to the gym is going to help her lose weight if her number one weakness is sugar. Eating too much sugar is far too damaging on her ass and her pancreas than can be fixed on the treadmill.

If sugar is your number one vice, your time would be better spent at the grocery store and in the kitchen planning meals ahead of time to curb your sweet tooth (more on how to do this shortly) than going to the gym.

Wake up, sit straight, snap out of it—start focusing on what will really get you results. Weight loss will happen quickly if you don't dilly dally on the minor things that are important for someone else but not important for you.

Have you identified your three biggest weaknesses and written them down? If you didn't do it a minute ago, do it now. The top three things you know are preventing you from losing weight. I'm sure you know what they are and don't have to think too hard. Here are some common areas people struggle with:

No willpower.

Don't know *what* to eat.

Hungry all the time.

No time to plan.

No time to cook.

Don't like to cook.

Eating late at night.

Eating too much in general.

Eating out too much.

Not getting enough exercise.

Eating too much sugar.

Eating when you're not hungry.

Eating too much candy.

Eating too many carbs, bread, pasta, beer, etc.

Eating out of social or familial obligation.

Drinking too much alcohol.

No time to cook healthy.

Don't like vegetables.

Don't like healthy foods in general.

Depressed and emotionally eating.

So? Which ones are your reasons? Don't see yours on there? Feel free to write it in—I left space. What is the number one thing you think is preventing you from losing weight? This is where you'll begin focusing your energy first.

Onward, we'll sift through the above concerns and other issues over the course of this book to try and help you navigate your way to your goal as quickly as possible. Only when you have a handle on your three biggest areas of weakness should you continue working your way through the wellness continuum. Remember that where you focus your efforts might be different than where so-and-so focuses their efforts, and it should be this way. Don't get sucked in to someone else's diet plan or workout routine that doesn't focus on your specific areas on concern.

Did I mention exercise sucks for weight loss?

I know, I know—you can't believe I said it.

Well, it does.

Abs are made in the kitchen not in the gym.

Buckle up. We're just getting started.

Chapter 3

"EXERCISE IS A TOUCHY LITTLE BITCH."

Do not count on exercise to lose weight. Exercise is good for you, no doubt. It's good for weight loss, too, if you commit to it every day. Or at least four days a week at an intensity and duration that will actually make a difference. But if you can't rev up your mojo to hit it like it's hot and you're counting on exercise to burn calories, you're screwed like the cork I just popped from my favorite bottle of wine.

If you think that lack of exercise is one of the pesky culprits preventing your weight loss, it's probably not. Go look over the list again. Not working out enough is not likely to be the reason you are not losing weight. Duh... *it's your diet!* What you eat or don't eat is infinitely more important for weight loss *and* overall health than exercise will ever be.

Exercise is a touchy little bitch.

Sometimes she helps you lose weight, and sometimes she strings you along, shows you her tits, and then laughs when you fall for her trick. But still, you pursue her, because she promises to give you a happy ending. She tells you to try harder, run faster, lift heavier. You believe her so you do it—until the next time you get on the scale and you've actually fucking gained weight.

If you've given up on working out to lose weight, I don't blame you. Working out is hard, and boring, and if you're not seeing or feeling the gains you expect, why continue? Finding the motivation to do something you don't want to do especially when you're not seeing results is really freaking difficult. Stupid, actually. What other activity would you devote so much time and effort toward without getting the results you want? Would you keep mowing the lawn, night after night, if the grass still wasn't getting any shorter and maybe, it was actually getting longer? No. You'd find another way to cut that shit down. I'd rent an industrial size bush whacker and give that thing a Brazilian.

So, if you're working out to lose weight and not losing weight—well, do I really have to finish this sentence? Let me rephrase, listen closely:

You can lose weight permanently by changing your

diet and not exercising—free pass.

You cannot lose weight permanently by exercising and not changing your diet—bummer.

I didn't say working out wasn't beneficial—of course it is. I also didn't say *not* to do it, of course you *should* do it. But statistically, you're probably not doing it and maybe never will. Or if you are doing it, you might not be doing it long and hard enough to get the results you desire anyway.

So let's re-think this. You don't like working out, or maybe you *do* like working out but just can't find the time; it doesn't produce the dramatic results that changing your diet does; so you're putting your energy into your workouts but not putting your energy into changing your diet because... why?

Here's where exercise *does* work for weight loss.

Let's say you weigh 150 pounds and your ideal weight is 135–140 pounds. If you've held steady at 150 pounds for as long as you can remember, adding in a few days a week of moderate intensity exercise, if you aren't already doing so, should get you to your goal and keep you there. But you'll have to keep at it. Forever. Or your weight will creep back up.

If this is you and all you have is 10 pounds to lose, don't worry about your diet. *Get your ass to the gym!* Changing your diet to keep those last few pounds off is harder than finding time to fit in regular exercise—trust me, I know. Saying no to every last morsel of food or alcohol that makes life enjoyable, sometimes merely tolerable, is nearly impossible, but that is exactly what it takes to keep those last few pounds off. For everyone else who has more than 10 pounds to lose and struggles to commit to regular exercise, you'd be wasting your time trying to exercise the weight away before making permanent changes to your diet first. Sure, you could sweat away 50 pounds, but if you haven't done the foundational ground work of changing how you think and what you eat, you'll gain it all back when you get injured and can't work out or when you simply can no longer find the willpower to get your ass to the gym.

It's not that exercise doesn't work because it does. The problem is our lack of commitment and consistency to it. Remember this: *Do not count on exercise to lose weight. Change your diet to lose weight. Then add in the type, intensity and duration of activity that you enjoy.* You'll be surprised that when the pressure is off of using exercise for weight loss how you might actually want to do it.

Some years ago, I found myself in a situation where I was required to eat my own advice. "Lose weight with your diet first," I'd been saying. "Get to where you want to be, or very close, *then* add in the kind of exercise you like, when you like to do it, so that when the inevitable comes and we all stop exercising for whatever reason, lazy, injury, boredom, vacation, it doesn't affect your weight. This way, when you *do* exercise, you can do it because you like it and want to, not because you think you have to. You won't ever have to worry about if you're burning enough calories if you don't count on burning those calories to lose weight."

Then, you can walk or pole dance or garden because you want to. If you prefer to play the guitar, paint, write, or doodle pictures of cats, then you are free to do as you wish without the fear of gaining weight while you sit all day.

I didn't say sitting all day is good for you—it's actually horrible for you, almost as bad as ingesting radioactive glow-in-the-dark sludge. It'll eat away at your spine.

Sitting is the new smoking, they say.

But if your passion (if you're one of the lucky

people who've actually figured out what your passion is) requires you to be sedentary, at least you won't gain weight doing it *if* you have your diet figured out. I have found myself on my ass more than any other time in my life while writing; but there is nowhere I'd rather be. I have to continually balance cellulite promoting activities with cellulite fighting activities.

I suppose every good adviser has to experience the advice they give. Yes, well I did. I was going along my merry way, my advice working for myself as intended, when I was forced to test it under the most extreme circumstances. I wrote about having a back injury in *AFFAIRYTALE*, and how it forced me into a sedentary lifestyle for years. I went from being immersed in a career where 10 plus hours a week of exercise was the minimum to nothing. Zilch. Walking was too active; zigzagging one city block became a treacherous feat of extreme agony that would end in me crawling home. Sneezing was so painful the internal pressure it produced felt like I was going to explode. From the time of injury through a behemoth back surgery and year of recovery, in all, I spent three years without even going for a walk. A real walk—zigzagging a block in a back brace doesn't count.

The nature of my ailment was an exercise-induced

overuse injury that resulted in ruptured disks and an 85 percent collapse in my lower spine. My vertebrate were sitting on top of one another grinding together when I moved. I could hear it. I wanted to kill myself. Thank God I didn't. I rather enjoy my life now after a truly miraculous surgery.

My point is, during that entire time from injury to recovery, I weighed 110–120 pounds, my usual fluctuation before two additional little people were heaved from my womb. I went from 10 or more hours a week of exercise to zero for three years and I did not gain one ounce of weight. Speculate all you want about my body's composition changing, but I didn't lose muscle or gain body fat as an even swap of weight, I tracked it—remember... obsessive dieter and chronic annoying overachiever.

Interestingly, the first few months when my injuries were so bad I had to stop moving, I actually lost weight. Not muscle weight either; I visibly had less body fat. It was as if my body had been sending my brain a signal that up until then was not getting through. The message was:

Stop fucking exercising. It's too much, you dumb shit. And if you don't listen, I'm going to give you an injury and make you listen.

Well, I didn't listen then, but I'm not as foolish now.

After surgery, I lay on my side for months, cried for months, lost my mind for months, and then I slowly picked up the broken pieces of my new life, while learning how to move my body in a way that didn't make it uninhabitable. I have since successfully continued to follow my self-imposed rule of not using exercise to lose weight.

It's taboo to talk about the negative impacts of exercise, I know—but I'll dabble in witchcraft for a moment anyway, because I think it's important. At first glance, the individuals who are in the gym every day for years, dedicated, proud they've never taken more than a day off here or there, would be someone to aspire to. However, upon further investigation, many of those many individuals who engage in that level of movement over a lifetime have a plethora of injuries—tendonitis, arthritis, general aches and pains with too early of an onset, bad knees, bad hips, etc. Not all, I said, but some.

In my early days as a young, green, personal trainer, I saw my share of women who had been avid exercise nuts. Most came to me with existing injuries, tears, sprains, aches, pains, early arthritis, stress fractures, etc., and I saw my share of women, of healthy weight who had rarely exercised in their lifetime but wanted to start now. These women were the population with little to no wear and tear. No injuries from decades of pavement pounding and joint-abusing activities.

Lest they worry! Because as trainers do, I immediately subjected them to the usual gauntlet of weight room and pavement-pounding activities to help them catch up to their already crippled counterparts. Until I wised up.

Now... before you throw your dumbbells at me, I feel I must say that I recognize the benefits of weight training, running, exercising in general, blah, blah, blah. Yes, there are benefits, more than can be written in one book, and yes, we should all be exercising. I like a good sweat just as much as anyone, but these days, I just prefer it happen under the covers at midnight.

There needs to be a new paradigm that doesn't exclude the hidden secrets of the exercise underground no one wants to talk about. Such as, exercise-induced injuries, excessive wear on your joints, repetitive overuse injuries, mineral depletion and generalized workout recommendations not appropriate for everyone that consequently can cause great injury to the types of bodies not suited.

Thank you, leg extension machine, for giving me chondromalacia so that when I get up from off the floor every time for the rest of my life, everyone knows I'm approaching and yells "the crack lady is coming!" And thank you, triceps pushups for engaging my overachieving mentality—you two have taken all the pleasure out of drinking a cup of coffee, since I can't even hold the fucking mug my tendonitis hurts so bad! Sometimes. I've worked for years to reverse the effects of exercise abuse on my body, and there is so much I wish I could take back.

Let's not forget weight gain. You can gain a shit ton of weight from having consistent, excessively high levels of cortisol which can happen from over exercising. If you're thinking, *well that certainly isn't me, I don't get enough exercise,* that is probably true, but don't be fooled, you do not need to be running marathons to be over exercising. Cortisol is released anytime the body feels stressed. Some exercise like walking, yoga or tai chi lowers cortisol while intense exercise several days a week for many months or years can cause excess cortisol which promotes abdominal fat gain, impairs your immune system and makes you dumber by decreasing your ability to think clearly.

"In the short term, stress can shut down appetite... But if stress persists—or is perceived as persisting—it's a different story. The adrenal glands release another hormone called cortisol, and cortisol increases appetite and may also ramp up motivation in general, including the motivation to eat. Once a stressful episode is over, cortisol levels should fall, but if the stress doesn't go away—or if a person's stress response gets stuck in the "on" position— cortisol may stay elevated." (Walter C. Willet 2012)

In conclusion, does this mean exercise is bad and you shouldn't do it? Yes, and no. It depends on how crazy nutso you are about it and the type of exercise you're doing. I was mental and went overboard. Now I'm smarter.

Burnout is real.

Over exercising is real.

Exercise for weight loss is overrated.

No amount of exercise will ever reverse the cheesecake that's clogging your arteries if your diet is the typical meat-eating American cuisine. No need to kill yourself in the gym if you're still putting pork on the grill—that'll get cha' regardless your efforts on the step mill.

Without excess movement, your joints have already sustained a lifetime of impact and torque. The more you move, the more your knees, hips, spine and every joint that articulates wears down. Some movement is good. It oils the joints, keeps you limber and can help negate the pain of arthritis. But too much causes more arthritis (inflammation of any joint) and eventually your bones say, *"fuck you I'm not going to move anymore"* and they grow together to prevent movement in that joint. That is the etiology of arthritis. It's terribly excruciating, irreversible and does not receive enough attention. If you haven't had arthritis and think it's an old person's disease that prevents them from opening tight lids off jars, you're right. What gets less attention is how severely debilitating arthritis can be in every joint at any age.

I have had clients not yet twenty with arthritis in their lower backs, elbows, hips and knees from a short but exuberant lifetime of exercise in less than two decades. Impact increases bone density and strengthens muscles, but not without a cost. To be fair, I've also met individuals who have regularly exercised moderately for decades and are fairly unscathed.

The best advice on exercise is this, do a little bit of everything, not too much of anything.

Did I mention I never run? Never. If a serial killer who was known for cutting up his victims and eating their eyeballs on crackers was chasing me, I would not run. It hurts and I'm sloth-like slow. Not everybody has a runner's body. For those of us who have big jugs, semi-knocked knees and limited mental endurance, all running does is cause stretched boobs, a serious knee or hip injury and wastes 45 minutes of time on something totally unenjoyable. Some bodies are perfectly designed for running and will never have issues with injury; others will never adapt without long term consequences. Find what works and what is actually healthy for your body.

I would advise walking. Not power walking or jogging—one could argue those are worse than running. Look it up.

Do yoga, but don't be stupid about it, and know your limits.

Learn Tai Chi.

Go hiking or kayaking or swimming.

Find a dance partner! If you can't then take off your clothes, put in Beyoncé and jiggle around yourself.

Did I mention walking?

Be easy on your joints.

Love your joints, don't injure them.

Find minimal impact activities if you want to preserve the health of your joints, keep cortisol levels low and your appetite under control. Don't run just because you think you need to; only run if you want to and it feels good. If it doesn't feel good, go find something that when you're done doing it, it does. Yes, push yourself—but not over a fucking cliff.

There are examples of people who have lost weight by going hog shit crazy working out, lots of them. Some keep it off for a lifetime, some gain it back. It is clearly possible to lose a mammoth amount of weight with exercise. If you have the courage and commitment to join that league of extraordinary humans, do it. If not, abandon the notion that working out will get you to your ultimate weight-loss goal if you have not been able to do it already.

Working out and not losing weight after you've tried it many times is like taking back your ex after he lied to you, cheated on you, and left you when you needed him most. Then when he begged to come back, you took him in because you thought this time would be different. Then he did it to you all over again.

You know what they say about taking back your ex,

don't you? It's like trying to put shit back in your asshole.

Chapter 4

WILLLPOWER:

noun | will·pow·er |\'wil-ˌpau̇(-ə)r\

1. the ability to control one's self

2. strong determination that allows you to do something difficult like not eat your child's leftovers

Never trust your willpower.

News flash: if you haven't had any before, you won't have any in the future. Has your willpower failed countless times like mine has? Do you have the strength to say no to the creamy dreamy chip dip at a New Year's party or the homemade fudge at Christmas? No? So why keep trying? Give up. Give in. Throw in the towel. So you have no willpower, so what? It doesn't really matter anyway. You don't need willpower to lose weight as long as you still have a brain.

If you're like me and at times have little to no self-control, then you have two choices. I suggest using a combination of both:

1. Avoid the situations where you know your willpower will fail.

2. Plan to be bad. Expect to eat like shit and plan for it ahead of time.

Avoid where you can, but know that you won't be able to avoid all social or familial obligations that revolve around food. Planning ahead, and anticipating that your willpower will fail, sets you up for success. If you have no willpower and you have to be somewhere with temptations you know you can't resist, don't even try to stay away from the frosted blue cupcakes and sugar-loaded bowl of frothy sorbet punch. Go ahead, have some, if that's what you like. Get it over with, and enjoy the party and the food. If you can't avoid it, you just have to plan for it ahead of time. Build in naughtiness.

You can be bad; you should be bad. But you have to pick and choose when you're going to be bad ahead of time, so it's not all the time.

If you have no willpower to exhibit proper portion control and you know you'll eat the entire pan of brownies, then for fuck's sake, don't bake them—avoid. Prevent putting yourself in any situation where you know you'll fail. If you want to lose weight, you must avoid certain situations where you can't say no.

If you know you have no willpower to exhibit proper portion control and you are going to make the brownies anyway, then just go ahead and fucking eat them. But don't be pissed when you can't eat anything else for three days after; you made the decision to eat rather than avoid. So go ahead, be bad; just be good in the days preferably before or after your dirty binge. And know that your good behavior has to be as extreme as the bad behavior or this will Never. Ever. Work.

If your past behavior is an indicator of your future choices, and there's a good possibility you'll eat the Oreos on top of the microwave while you're making dinner, don't bring them into the house. If they are already in your house, you have two choices.

1. Get rid of them. Destroy them quick, close your eyes and give them a cold shower.

2. Eat them, but know that like charging a few hundred dollars on your credit card, now you can't charge anything for the rest of the week. You had your binge, and

now you have to pay off your debt. Better yet, get one of those credit cards where you can only spend whatever amount of money you've put on it ahead of time. Then you won't have any debt to repay. Do you get me? Be really good, so you can be bad when you really need to.

Think of it this way, would you set yourself up for failure in any other situation? Would you take your little kids to the beach for the day without packing enough snacks to feed an army? Fuck no, they'd eat you alive in the first hour. Plan to be bad when you know you will be.

If you have a friend or spouse who needs you as their co-dependent eater and can't just go get ice cream on their own—they have to drag everyone else down with them—ditch them. If you can't, then engage that person in a different activity. Ask if they want to go to the park instead or go for a walk or pick mushrooms, whatever.

The hubs and I usually go out to eat once a week— alone. This is significant—one or two hours alone with my husband each week. We make time, Grandma watches the kids, and we defend our date night as if it were our first born. We drink, we laugh, make sexual innuendos, tell distasteful jokes, and by the end of our date night, we've solved all the world's problems—if only someone would listen to our ideas.

Most often when we go out we eat just the salad bar because we both *want* to eat healthy and feel good when we do. We've made it a mutual goal in which we support each other, most of the time.

However, one of us may not always feel like being healthy on date night. Perhaps one of us has skipped lunch and might eat a small child if food doesn't arrive soon, or perhaps one of us has had an extra spectacular day and just wants to celebrate—and who celebrates with a salad bar and lemon water?

I plan for this date night each week by making it my assumed cheat night. I plan on the hubs holding his stomach and trying not to burst out laughing when we make eye contact because he knows that I know he's setting the stage to ask me if I want to split a lavash (basically a pizza but with a flakey cracker crust topped with Havarti cheese and loads of vegetables) and I always do. Other times he wants just the salad bar, but I'm the lead criminal begging him, rationalizing and bargaining for him to eat dirty with me.

Sometimes our weeks get out of hand and one lavash week with double the drinks spills over into the next four weeks. At which point, I feel I need to redirect that path we're on because I'm encroaching on my self-imposed upper weight limit.

So I try this:

"Honey, let's hit the gym tonight instead of going out." Which is usually me with enthusiasm for about 10 seconds.

Then he says "Nah... we want to go to our favorite place, right?"

To which I reply by raising my voice and index finger. "OK, but we're not having a bread board, and we're not ordering lavash. We have to eat salad bar. Promise?" I hold out my pinky. And he promises. So we are back on the salad bar kick for at least another five weeks before one of us dares to lead the other back down the path of gluttony and drunkenness.

But, each week I plan to fail by assuming that I'll cave in to another drink and cheese and crackers instead of the salad bar. As long as I plan for it and make it my cheat night, regardless if it happens or not, my weight is generally unaffected. All of this means that I have to say no to anything else that comes up in the week that involves eating out. If I don't adhere, I don't stay skinny. And I like being skinny more than I like eating out more than once a week.

My client Sandy, when I asked her what food or situation she couldn't resist she said, "Pizza is an asshole. I love him and hate him." Now there is a woman who can admit she loves an asshole. Sandy has even admitted to waking up with his sauce on her face and not remembering the roll in the sheets that got it there. She is weak to him and she knows it.

That's the best part about Sandy. She is aware of her asshole addiction. Now she's is in a position of power to control her love affair with Mr. Secret Sauce. Most of the time, Sandy can control how often she comes in to contact with him. She can, more often than not, choose not to be in the same room with him; chose not to allow him to hang with her and her obnoxious friends. She can certainly choose not to keep his leftovers lying around the house. When she's stuffed full of him and wants him to leave, while she still has strength, she throws him away—she knows she has to, so she does, and that's a crucial part of her pact with herself.

What Sandy can't control, unfortunately, is when she's in an inebriated state and he is her booty call. Not once, not twice, more times than she'd like to admit—she has made that shameful call to Papa John that she doesn't remember in the morning. In fact, the only reason she even knows he came over is because his sauce was still on the sheets.

But Sandy has figured this problem out, too. She knew she was going out on Friday night with her good time girls and might slosh back a few too many margaritas, thus opening up the potential for her to make the booty call later. So during the week, Sandy avoided contact with all the other assholes in her life. Then when Friday night came, she could partake in the beverages of her choice and have her booty call, too. Friday night was the only time that week she'd been bad. One night, one meal, one food. It doesn't affect her total weight loss. She can still lose two to three pounds most weeks with one bender planned in. But just one—for Sandy, but that might be different for you. It's up to you to determine how naughty you can be and still make progress.

I prefer to sprinkle my bender around. I need room to eat like I need room to breathe. I need to be a little bad every day not just one day a week. I cheat a little every day and know that I can have one cheat evening in addition to that and still *maintain* my weight. If I want to lose, I have to tighten up the apron strings. This is just my personal preference, and it is part of the plan I've created for myself through trial and error and the study and observation of me.

Next, my client whose name rhymes with Schmericka. She has a weakness that comes served on a warm platter with crispy, salty, tortilla chips and ooey-gooey cheese. It's a dish well-traveled; she nearly can't avoid it. Wait for it... spinach and artichoke dip.

Which, ironically, sounds healthy but any idiot knows the majority of the contents are butter and cheese. She has also admitted her weakness for straight-up cheese, cut into different geometrical shapes, breaded and fried, served with ranch and marinara, mixed together.

Bubbling hot goo cannot be a part of her regular weight maintenance routine if she wants to keep fitting into her size threes. So she has figured out how much she can cheat and who she really likes to rendezvous with, so she never gets caught with her pants down and not able to pull them back up.

The face of evil is fried cheese, yes, but this demon is easy to banish if you know how to exorcise him. Here is the conversation that my friend whose name rhymes with Schmericka had with her conscience so that she can live a long skinny life in washed-out size threes.

Schmericka: I will say no to artichoke dip, cheese

curds or mozzarella sticks when I go out. I will eat dinner before I go, so that when I get there, I'm not hungry. I have the willpower to say no. I can do it.

Conscience: Sorry, bitch, no you can't. You've never been able to do it before, so why would I believe you now?

Schmericka: How dare you?! OK, go fuck yourself, you're right. Who am I kidding, of course I can't say no.

Conscience: Find something to cut out elsewhere. You must make a sacrifice.

Schmericka: So I can have artichoke dip tonight with drinks at the bar as long as I sacrifice something of equal value elsewhere?

Conscience: Give me food or give me sweat!

Schmericka: I'll give you sweat! I'll work out for three hours tomorrow. I swear.

Conscience: You and I both know your ass won't make it to the gym. And even if it does, there ain't no way it'll be there for three hours. It must be a food sacrifice!

Schmericka: Fine.

Conscience: May your soul be happy and your thighs skinny.

Are cheat days OK?

Not only are they OK, they are necessary.

Figure out how much you want to and *can* cheat.

Build it in.

Will you still lose weight?

Of course, if you are using them as they are intended and have figured out how many times you can have an affair and not get caught. Maybe you can only indulge one day a week, or only one meal a week; only you can figure this out. Maybe you need to cheat a little every day when no one's looking, like me. Maybe you have no weekend willpower so you have to be extra good all week because Saturday and Sunday are your cheat days. Figure out what works for you.

A word of caution: two full cheat days over the weekend will likely stop your weight loss. I don't know many people who can do this and still stay lean besides my brother who otherwise eats a super strict diet Monday–Friday. Countless times I've weighed clients in on a Monday morning at 135 pounds then on Friday they weigh in at 133 pounds. After the weekend, on Monday morning, they are 135 pounds again and the cycle continues until they figure out how to get their weekend under control. Which means different things to different people.

Prioritize what you really like and what you can pass up. You might try rating things on a scale of one to ten, ten being "*I have zero willpower against it,*" and one being "*Meh... I can do without.*" Only eat eights, nines and tens. Or just nines and tens. This might not be setting you up for preventing colorectal cancer, but at least you won't be gaining weight over the weekend.

Weight loss isn't science, it's art. Well, it's a little of both, but the art part of it is subjective and must be tailored to you. It's tricky to figure out how many cheat meals or days or treats you can get away with. Especially if your lifestyle and schedule changes dramatically from week to week. There are always going to be factors that are constant and factors that are constantly changing. You'll have to be flexible and experiment like you did in college. Your cheat schedule should look unique and be built around the foods, meals, social and familial situations, and days of the week in which you *know* you have little or no willpower to overcome.

One more important thing here—anticipate there are going to be events that are out of your control *every week*, events that you didn't expect. Let's say you forgot about your friend's birthday, whoops. And everyone typically convenes at a classy restaurant, eats, and indulges in a several bottles of vino. You didn't plan for this, oh wait you did! You planned for the unplanned because you knew something always comes up, so you were good all week knowing there would be *something* unavoidable where you had no willpower.

Assume that at least one or more times a week you'll have to call an audible and change the play. You can either avoid or plan for the unplanned. Or both.

Chapter 5

CALORIE:

noun | cal·o·rie [kal-uh-ree]

plural: *calories*

1. a unit equal to the kilocalorie, used to express the heat output of an organism and the fuel or energy value of food

2. tiny creatures who live in your closet that sew your clothes a little bit tighter each night

"...people in countries where obesity is extremely rare, like China, eat substantially more calories (2,630 kcals a day) than the obesity capital of the world, America (2,360 kcals)." (Holford 2006)

How can this be? I'm so confused!

Actually, I'm not. It's very easy really... because a calorie is not a calorie.

This is important.

A calorie is the amount of energy needed to raise the temperature of one kilogram of water by one degree Celsius. Blah, blah, blah... WTF does that mean?

It means that a calorie is determined from a reaction that happens inside a test tube of water. No matter the source it is derived from (carbohydrate, protein or fat) a calorie is a calorie... *in a test tube.*

In your body, those three stooges have very different impacts. And it's never about intent; it's always about impact.

The problem with the calorie theory is that your stand-in body double, the test tube, fails to accurately replicate the millions of physiological reactions that happen in your body. For those of us who are more complex than test tubes, this is a problem.

I could tell you all the bazillion functions of proteins which basically remodel your entire body every decade or so. Then elaborate on how fat also has a gazillion purposes not the least of which is being a membrane in every cell in your 32 trillion cell body. We could discuss all the kinds of carbohydrates and what is good or bad but that's all quite boring, and you can go look it up if you want to know those things. None of those functions and outcomes are replicated in the calorie test tube experiment.

Here's what you need know:

Even though they act the same in a test tube, a calorie of carbohydrate acts differently in your body than a calorie of protein; a calorie of protein acts differently than a calorie of fat; vice versa, so-on-and-so-forth. Got it? Good.

The calorie theory assumes that all calories have an equal impact when they enter your body, and thus, the outcome is predictable and measurable. Calories in— 1,200, calories out—1,700, easy, measurable, quantifiable. At this rate, if you did this every day, by the end of one week you'd be two pounds lighter. If you did this a second week you'd be another two pounds lighter. At the end of six months you would be 48 pounds lighter. Wow, sounds foolproof. Well... go ahead and try it. Eat whatever you want—1,200 calories in donuts at 10 p.m. naked in your bathtub—and see if you'll still lose weight.

Wait... don't try that. For two reasons:

1. Because it's a program, a system—a method that you'll follow as religiously as you have tried to in the past—but at some point, you'll fall off.

2. The calorie theory is fundamentally flawed. Weight loss can be, unfortunately, much more psychologically and physiologically complex than calories in, calories out.

Even when "healthy" choices are encouraged on a calorie counting regime the definition of what's healthy is subjective and depends on who thinks what is healthy. Are 100 calorie snack packs of cookies, low fat pretzels or other low calorie, low fat food-like items healthy? Depends on who you ask. What about weight loss shakes, protein bars, liquid meal replacements? Do you consider those healthy?

Like global warming, "healthy" has become a phenomenon where people take sides rather than look at the evidence or think critically about the problem. And in nutrition, religion and politics, it seems that everyone believes what they want to believe regardless of the evidence.

So, what is healthy? I certainly have my opinions on this issue and would like to think they are rooted in the evidence based on epidemiologic observations of populations of people, their lifestyle, their diet and their incidence of disease. But whatever I think is healthy, there will certainly be a good argument against it as well, so I've given up on defining "healthy." I do what is right and feels good for me and my family and what keeps me skinny and free from heart disease. This means not paying attention to calories, rather eating whole food, mostly plants.

Calories matter when the food you're considering is something you know will cause you to gain weight or that you suspect is "unhealthy." Like sugar-loaded coffee drinks or pan pizza. Put these no-brainer, high-calorie choices into perspective by playing *would you rather.* Traditionally, the game would go something like this...
Would you rather lick the bottom of a homeless person's bare foot or eat a live goldfish? Would you rather eat your husband's toenail clippings or lick the rim of a public toilet seat? Now those are tough choices. Playing the game with food and exercise is much less disgusting but still motivates you to make the right choice.

Would you rather eat two slices of pizza and have to run on the treadmill for two hours OR would you rather have dinner at home before you go to the pizza place?

Would you rather eat one jumbo muffin and weight train for 75 minutes OR buy the fresh cut fruit next to it and get fucking skinny while eating it?

Pay attention to the mammoth number of calories

that are in undisputed unhealthy foods. Remind yourself what you would have to do to burn those calories off. Google it.

Don't worry about how many calories are in black bean chili or how many grams of sugar is in a banana. Forget that someone told you not to eat avocados or watermelon. Does it really make sense to cut those things out and eat chicken instead?

Whole plant foods are what will keep you skinny and disease free. If you dig deep enough into the pit of your stomach and ask it if this is true... the answer to *WTF should I eat?* has been there all along.

Plants.

Mostly plants.

Drink wine, eat plants.

Eat all the whole plant foods you like. You will never have to count calories on a *mostly* plant diet. Over a lifetime, whole plant foods will keep you skinny and healthy regardless of their calories.

With that, I will not be making specific calorie recommendations, or recommendations of grams of this or that. It's an outdated, reductionist way of thinking about health and weight loss. For too long food science has been reducing food into its smallest components then determining how much of what we should eat based on that. Rather than simply picking up a peach that we innately know is the right choice—duh.

The notion that we have to meticulously track calories or grams of fat or protein in everything we eat is ludicrous. If you eat a diet of mostly plants you won't have to worry about tracking anything to stay healthy and skinny.

The food environment we live in has spoon-fed us to believe that we are not capable by ourselves of making sound choices about what to put in our mouths. Since we are incompetent to make our own choices then, food manufacturers have created a profitable system where they conduct studies that tell us precisely what foods to eat and in what amounts. You wouldn't trust a teacher who was "teaching" you about nutrition and at the same time selling you their nutritional products and making billions, would you? Something smells rancid about this.

Don't use calories to determine what to eat, use your brain. Your common sense, how your clothes fit, how much energy you have, how you look naked, the scale, your blood pressure, your cholesterol, the strength of your immunity against illness. All of these factors will tell you what is healthy and what is not.

But, if you're making bad choices because you are choosing to, or you just can't say no, then counting calories may give you boundaries you cannot give to yourself. In this case, fine, go ahead, use it as a tool.

But there is a better way.

Eat plants.

Mostly plants.

Drink wine, eat plants.

I'll address the iron and other deficiency concerns shortly. Wait, no I won't—because there aren't any. Anything you get from animal foods you can get and absorb much better from plants. You're not a carnivore, your dog is. Your intestines are made for digesting plants, and Fido's innards are made for digesting meat.

You were prepared for that scolding right? I warned you I'd sprinkle some plant-eating propaganda in here.

...

I've been consulting and speaking on different weight-loss and wellness topics for almost two decades (I was seventeen when I had my first gig. I suppose you're doing the math to see how old I am. If I look younger than 37 on the cover photo, I blame it on plants, Botox, and wine.) After each speech, there is a line of questions which I'm happy to indulge. One common question sticks out because of the desperate voice and frustrated eyes that almost always accompany it:

I've been eating healthy, I swear it, and I'm still not losing weight. Could it be that I'm not eating enough calories?

If you don't eat enough food, you'll lose weight and eventually die—this is certain. There has not been a case where someone has emerged from a starvation situation plump and proclaimed, "I just wasn't eating enough calories so I didn't lose any weight."

What your body does, is go into a "starvation mode." It's called *adaptive thermogenesis.* When you reduce calorie intake, your body responds by decreasing calorie expenditure. Life's a bitch, ain't it? You're working hard at making good choices and resisting temptations all the while there's some bitch inside the control room making sure you'll never be successful.

70

When that wench feels like your making progress, she turns down the metabolic dial one notch at a time, trying her best to keep you fat. However, if I fell off a cliff while hiking in Yosemite and lived, I'd apologize for calling her names. Because I understand that she has a sworn duty to save my life by turning down my metabolism to conserve energy and keep me alive while I'm waiting to be rescued.

When you cut calories, this broad in the control room senses it almost immediately. So, the answer to the desperate question is—yes, it could be that you are not eating enough calories and that is why you are not losing weight. If you cut calories enough, eventually you'll lose weight no doubt—it's a damn quagmire. You'll have to ask yourself if cutting calories until you get low enough to lose weight is sustainable for you.

For me, cutting calories ends in utter disaster. If I intentionally cut too many calories, I've instantly sounded the alarms, awoken the sleeping witch, and engaged in a broom fight I'll never win. She will always win, her soul purpose is to keep me alive and her determination has far more endurance than what I have to adhere to a very low calorie diet.

I need to be able to eat the house down and the

garage too, *if I want to*. And I can do that, and still stay skinny, only if I eat whole plant foods. You know... fruits, nuts, vegetables, lentils, beans.

Instead of cutting calories and engaging her in a game you'll never win, on her turf, instead you *can* out maneuver her. Stick with eating a diet of *mostly* plant foods. Eat all the whole plant foods you want (I've included recipes.) Doing so will not cut your calorie intake substantially enough to sound any alarms. Eventually, the control freak behind your eyes will realize that you're not trying to put her out of a job, and she'll slowly speed you up again.

If for some unknown reason she decides to put on the breaks and turn your metabolic fires down, sit tight, hold your course, steady now. Eat all the plants you want, she'll eventually realize you're eating enough calories and turn the dial back up.

Remember, different types of foods affect weight loss differently, so whereas eating 2,300 calories of crap will forever make you gain weight, eating 2,300 calories of whole plant foods will keep you losing and will keep the broad with all the metabolic power happy.

People have success busting through weight-loss

plateaus by tricking this adaptive mechanism with high-calorie days. They are not only glorious; they fool your 200,000-year-old biology into thinking there's plenty of food, so therefore, there is no need to conserve all that fat. You can't have high-calorie binge days every day, but when they do happen, they are actually beneficial.

The one thing I know about myself through trial and error, lots of it, is that when I am set on losing a few pounds, maybe five, maybe 10, it takes a while for my body to pick up what I'm laying down and produce results.

It's as if that chick in the control room knows I'm trying to shed a few pounds for my niece's wedding, and she'll be damned if she's going to let any of those lifesaving fat stores go. But with persistence, not too much cutting out, and increasing whole real plant foods, as long as I don't do anything too drastic, she forgets I'm trying to lose weight and turns up the juice again. Then voilà—10 or 15 pounds gone.

Be patient. I've had to be disciplined for many weeks with no results, knowing that eventually they'll come. They always do; sometimes it just takes a little while.

Chapter 6

"EATING LATE AT NIGHT IS THE SINGLE
MOST DETERMINTAL THING YOU CAN DO
TO SABBOTOGE YOUR WEIGHT LOSS."

By late at night, I don't mean eleven o'clock. I mean after dinner—an early dinner like 6 p.m. Yep. Six...ish.

If you were counting calories, *when* you eat your calories shouldn't matter as long as you don't exceed your total calorie allotment for the day, right? Well... try it. Eat your calories at night, see what happens.

The civilized communities of nutrition experts say that although it's not a great idea to eat late at night, it won't affect the scale as long as you stay under your allotted calories. I disagree, and since I'm more of a non-civilized heathen, I'll say that it most certainly does.

If you're one of those rare super heroes whose power is will and you can actually follow sensible eating instructions for snacking at night such as, stick to no more than one hundred calories (like 20 baby carrots) good for you. I have no such willpower.

If I am going to eat late at night, chances are I'm punch-drunk and not interested in raw vegetables. I'm looking for something naughty and exciting that will make me feel satisfied and want to fall asleep. Since I know this about myself, I have to plan accordingly earlier that day. That means being on my best behavior knowing that alcohol *can* decrease my ability to make good food decisions after 8 p.m.

Eating late at night is not only a sure way to stop weight loss but to put weight on no matter what you eat during the day. I'll go so far as to say *it doesn't matter what you eat all day, if you're eating late at night, you'll gain weight.* Conversely, I believe the opposite is true. *It doesn't matter what you eat all day, if you aren't eating late at night (after six...ish) you'll lose weight.*

If you have ever whined and said *I don't know why I'm not losing weight, I'm eating healthy,* provided that is actually true, one of the tricks you could try is to change nothing except be done with your food day at 6 p.m. or at least a few hours earlier than you were previously. But don't be an idiot and binge just before your cut-off time—

that would be self-sabotage.

Naomi eats an exceptionally clean diet, primarily plants, even though she is not a vegetarian or a vegan. Seemingly doing everything correct, she was struggling to lose weight at the bewilderment of us both. Short of resorting to a 500 calorie a day starvation diet and some bullshit like pray the fat away, she decided on her own that she would change nothing except she would stop eating every day at 4 p.m. That is freaking early and I have never recommended it. Not that it wouldn't work, it would just have a high failure rate. But if it behooves you to try, good luck. Prior to this change, Naomi was not eating after 7 p.m. but was still not able to budge the scale. She went to bed each night by 9 p.m., I think mostly to curb the temptation of eating.

However undesirable not eating after 4 p.m. is, it worked. She didn't decrease her calories or change what she ate; she ate sensibly. The only factor she changed was that all of the food she would normally eat over the course of the day, she consumed it now by 4 p.m. (One could argue that not eating for half a day decreases the total number of calories she consumed, but in this scenario, as I've said that was not the case.) She was able to lose those last stubborn 15 pounds and is now svelte with zero cottage cheese on her ass whatsoever—I can't say the same for myself. Boohoo.

So why the weight-loss success with not eating late in the day? I don't presume to know exactly *why* it worked, I just know it worked for her and others who have been brave enough to try it and strong enough to stick with it.

I speculate that since she fasted 14 hours each night before she "broke-the-fast" in the morning, this period of complete rest was what her body needed. There is nothing nefarious about fasting overnight for 12–14 hours if you are a healthy person. There are tremendous benefits to be gained from nightly fasting and juice fasting (which we'll discuss later). The rewards of allowing your body a daily period of long rest without eating food are nothing short of glorious. *If* you can do it.

"A sensible daily plan mixes fasting with eating. Each day can include 12–14-hour period of fasting from early evening through the night, as indeed breakfast was given that name to denote the time where we *break the fast* of the night," says Elson M. Haas, M.D. in his book *The Detox Diet*.

In order to pull off not eating after 6 p.m. or 4 p.m. or whenever you decide, consider a few things:

1. If you haven't eaten enough or smartly enough throughout the day, it will be impossible to overcome cravings at night.

If you've gotten yourself into this scenario, the way out of it is to find a distraction, go to sleep, or eat something and start over tomorrow without being such a dumb ass.

2. If you are thinking about food after dinner, ask yourself if you're actually hungry? If the answer is yes, eat enough during the day (not crap) to prevent this in the future. If the answer is no, then you'll need to look a bit deeper into your soul to find out why.

Consider that you're eating when you're not hungry because you're bored or unhappy or both. In this case, perhaps you could find a ritual. Something you can do each night that is satisfying for your belly and your mind. I drink tea. Special tea. Not just the crumbs left over after the real tea leaves have been harvested. I buy the real shit, so it's fun and special when I drink it. I like to buy teas from Special Teas Inc.

OK, I lied! I don't drink tea at night. I drink wine. But if for some rare reason I'm not drinking wine, I drink tea.

Then get yourself a special mug, cup it with both hands, and snuggle on the couch with a soft blanky. When it's a special ritual you like, you'll want to do it. Only then will it work to occupy the space where eating used to be.

If you don't like tea, create your own ritual; squeeze lemons, get an adult coloring book, watch porn, do a DIY project, get lost on Pinterest, whatever keeps you distracted and happy.

There are plenty of other emotionally fulfilling things to do with your life than peruse the kitchen until your willpower fails and you pig out. You just have to take the time to think about what they might be and write them down so you don't forget. Make a list of things that make you happy that you can do instead of eating.

Get out a piece of paper, and at the top of the page write, "*Things that make me happy.*" When you catch yourself thinking or looking for food after dinner and decide that it's not because you're actually hungry, say something like, "*I like being skinny more than I like eating after dinner.*" Then pick something from your list to occupy your mind and don't hesitate.

Here are some of the things on my list:

- Walk the dog

- Read a book

- Write

- ~~Meditate with mala~~

- Do yoga

- ~~Go to the gym~~

- Watch Netflix

- Watch *Game of Thrones*

- Wonder why I keep watching *Game of Thrones*

- Learn to make a new food

- Bust out the juicer

- Take a community class

- Teach a community class

- Go back to college

- Go visit someone

- Teach the dog a new trick

- ~~Teach the kids how to play the piano~~

- ~~Learn how to read notes~~

- ~~Learn how to play guitar~~

- Drink wine at sunset

- Drink wine and write down all the words that describe it

- Drink wine and get drunk

- Make a list of words I like

- ~~Clean the house~~

- ~~Organize the Tupperware~~

- ~~Do a DIY project~~

As I've fine-tuned my list, I've crossed off the items that no longer make me happy or have a tendency to make me angry. Put some time into figuring out the small things in life that make you happy. Do them instead of eating.

Back to Naomi. Perhaps she lost weight not because of a long daily rest from food but because she was getting adequate sleep. Which is *required* for but often overlooked as a key factor for weight loss.

The National Sleep Foundation states that, "Research has shown that too little sleep results in daytime sleepiness, increased accidents, problems concentrating, poor performance on the job and in school, and possibly, increased sickness and weight gain."

How much sleep do you need? Adults: 7-9 hours/night. Remember when your mom used to yell at you on the weekends if you slept in too late. Turns out that teenagers need more sleep, Mom—see, I wasn't just lazy, I was growing.

Just as important as getting enough sleep is getting quality sleep. Well… moms and dads out there with kids under four, you're fucked—might as well stay fat and cranky until the kids get a little older because it's damn impossible to get a restful night sleep with a gaggle of toddlers in the house after midnight. It's a helluva miracle I lost all the baby weight after each one of my three were born considering the chronic interrupted nights of sleep.

The good news, toddler moms and dads of the world, is that you're in the worst shape of your life right now. I can't think of a worse time to try to lose weight than with little kids in the house. Hang tight, you'll get through it, they will become more independent and when they do, you'll get skinnier.

Sleep is an ornery curmudgeon with an absurd amount of control over your weight loss. Not enough zzzs will stop your fat from wiggling out of its cells. Plenty of zzzs will help your body release a little hormone called leptin. Leptin and ghrelin (pronounced *greh-lin*) are the "hunger hormones."

When released:

- Leptin suppresses your appetite

- Ghrelin increases it

Both are creatures of the night, lurking around and waiting for their fetish to arrive—sleep. Leptin only comes out when you get enough sleep. He is not interested in you being fat or depressed; he wants you to look your best and helps you do that by suppressing your appetite all the next day.

But... Leptin only comes out to play if you get enough sleep, and to make matters worse, he requires that it be quality sleep too. If you don't, he'll punish you like the submissive you are and won't make an appearance the next day to suppress your appetite and help you get skinny. Only if you are deep sleeping at the witching hour will he bestow the magical gift of no appetite upon you.

If you become sleep deprived, Leptin will not come around. Instead, you'll get his slap-happy, booze-breath brother Ghrelin in your bedroom at night, and he'll get to have his way with you.

Ghrelin will bring a paddle and whip. His goal is to keep you fat and cut down your self-esteem by making you insatiably hungry. Ghrelin has the power to increase your appetite whenever he comes around and all the next day. But you have the power to keep Ghrelin away and have Leptin instead.

Get enough sleep, get a visit from Leptin, get skinny.

Get sleep deprived, get a visit from Ghrelin, get fat.

Would you rather go to bed early, get enough sleep, be made love to softly and encouraged gently? Or go to bed late each night and get nailed by a drunken sailor with a splintered paddle?

The benefits of adequate sleep for weight loss cannot be underestimated. If you are struggling to lose weight and truly are "eating healthy" just like stopping your food day at six, you might also consider changing nothing except getting enough quality sleep.

Now...

Are you sitting down?

Breakfast is not the most important meal of the day.

Chapter 7

"YOU CAN FIND A STUDY TO SUPPORT EITHER SIDE
OF EVERY ISSUE THAT HAS EVER EXISTED
SINCE THE BEGINNING OF TIME."

Breakfast is not the most important meal of the day. Lunch is. There, I said it. Whew! But don't tell my mother or she'll think she failed to instill anything sensible in me.

So *why* is breakfast the most important meal of the day? Because it jumpstarts your metabolism? Of course it does! That's why it's called *break-the-fast*. But does that mean you lose the benefits of breaking-the-fast if you don't eat your breakfast before a certain time? Fuck no. What if my breakfast is at 10 a.m. instead of 7 a.m.? Am I losing out on the purported benefits of breakfast because I fasted longer?

No.

Let's say I last ate at 8 p.m., went to bed at 11 p.m., then had toast with peanut butter at 8 a.m. That's a 12 hour overnight fast. Is that a better scenario than waiting until 10 a.m. (when I'm actually hungry) and having a 14 hour fast?

I'd prefer to break my fast when I'm actually hungry. And in doing so, for me, it actually reduces the amount of food I consume over the course of the day. When you're 5'4" and want to fit into a bikini, every morsel counts. The years of my life that I spent feeling so dirty and despicable for not eating breakfast are over. I've forced myself to eat breakfast more times than I have hair follicles and what I've found is, for me, it increases the total amount of food I eat in that particular day. Over the course of time, I gain weight for food I didn't even want to fucking eat.

Breakfast has been touted as a way to prevent diabetes, heart disease, and my favorite, eat breakfast = lose weight. The studies that have been done on these factors are not enough to convince me that if my clients or I start eating breakfast as the only thing we change in our lifestyles, we'll lose weight.

A July 2013 study in the journal *Obesity* reported that people who ate breakfast as their largest meal of the day lost an average of 17.8 pounds over three months in comparison to people who consumed the same number of total calories per day but ate most of their calories at dinner. The dinner group lost an average of 7.3 pounds per person (Jakubowicz, et al. 2013). A more digestible version of the study can be found via ScienceDaily.com under the title "Eating a big breakfast fights obesity and disease."

So what does this tell us? It tells *me* that eating late at night will make you gain weight no matter how many calories you consume during the day. My mind didn't make the leap that eating a big breakfast was the reason the first group lost more weight—they just didn't eat those calories at dinner or late at night when your body is naturally slowing down its processes, preparing you to get a restful night of uninterrupted sleep so Leptin can pay you a visit and make you skinny.

Is breakfast the most important meal of the day for helping you lose weight? Only if you don't eat a big dinner? But what if you do—where is that factor considered? I'd like to investigate a study that changed absolutely nothing in a person's diet *except* that they started eating a big breakfast and then lost weight because of that one factor alone. Can't find it.

I'm sure you'll find a study now and might even send it to my inbox—try and be polite. But you can find a study to support either side of every single issue that has ever existed since the beginning of time. I can't find anything *compelling enough* to convince me that breakfast is more important than lunch or dinner for weight loss. If you have been fasting for 12–14 hours and need to *break-the-fast*, that is when breakfast is damn important.

Is it OK to skip breakfast and not eat until lunch presents itself? It's clear that kids who don't eat breakfast have a harder time concentrating in school. But you are not a kid and you should have enough sense to know that if you are not mentally functioning at your best in the morning after you haven't had breakfast, then you should eat breakfast. If you are working out in the morning, you should eat breakfast; if you are just plain hungry at breakfast, eat breakfast.

But what if you're not hungry? Should you force yourself to eat breakfast anyway just to "jump start your metabolism?" How's that working for ya'—are you losing weight just because you're eating breakfast?

There are two types of non-breakfast eaters. The individuals who don't eat breakfast and binge later in the day because they've waited too long to eat and now they can't control themselves; if you're one of them, then eat breakfast, dummy, so you don't binge later. And the individuals who don't eat breakfast until they are hungry and don't binge later. If you're one of them, don't worry about forcing yourself to eat because you think you should. You'll be fine; your body is well-equipped for you to fast for long periods.

When you decide to break-the-fast, your body will respond accordingly and turn up your metabolic fires so you can finish your day.

Let yourself wake up and get hungry. If that means you're ready to eat at 9 a.m. instead of 7 a.m., eat at 9 a.m. If you're not hungry 'til 11 a.m., eat then. If you are working out, lifting weights or doing other physical activity a few days a week, you should eat at least 30 minutes before or right after your workout for optimal energy and recovery.

Let me be clear: I'm not telling you not to eat breakfast if you're hungry for breakfast. What I'm saying is that if you're not hungry for breakfast, it's OK to wait until you are. Eat when you're ready because breakfast is not the most important meal of the day.

Neither is dinner.

Mom yelled at my brother and me to not eat before dinner. She would slap crackers out of our hands and take away food so we wouldn't ruin our appetites. Today, she might be flabbergasted to know that I serve all three of my children a hearty snack before dinner every night I can.

I mostly do this so they leave me the hell alone and get out of the kitchen so I can cook dinner and drink wine in peace for fifteen minutes. The greater benefit of feeding them a snack before dinner is that they're not having a meltdown after not eating since lunch seven hours earlier. It seems to me that making them wait another hour after they've already been waiting seven is cruel.

If they eat before dinner, they get along, no one is cranky. Well... someone is always cranky—sometimes it's me. Letting them eat a bit before dinner buys me some extra time so I can get something halfway decent on the table.

I lied. We don't use the table. The table is really dusty. In fact, I'm getting rid of the table and putting in something that'll get used—a wine bar, right next to the piano, with red barrel chairs and a champagne chandelier. Now *that* will get used. Our kitchen table will forever be the island, sitting on barstools with our phones out and the T.V. on while the dog begs the two-year-old for food.

Which she obliges as she's watching *Frozen* and eating peas.

Lunch is the most important meal of the day. If all you had was a yogurt and an orange for lunch because you are trying to *eat light*, you've been duped. So you've had a late breakfast, now you'll have a late lunch, say 2 p.m. Make that lunch substantial, so that when 6 p.m. rolls around, you won't binge on dinner.

Eating a big dinner, no matter the time, is never a good idea for weight loss. The cycle of the human body is to begin slowing down in the late afternoon to prepare you for bed. So don't consume the majority of your calories during a time when your body is naturally slowing down. Slower metabolic rate = less energy burned = more body fat stored.

Want to lose weight?

Eat breakfast when you get hungry for it.

Make lunch the biggest meal of the day.

Taper down at dinner.

Don't eat after dinner.

I suppose you're ready to hear about *what* to eat

rather than *how* to eat... hold tight; there is one more important thing to discuss before we talk about specific food. If you get this one thing right, you will sail into the golden harbor of Skinny Town without ever being hungry again.

Chapter 8

HANGRY:

Adj. | han·gry | (hang-gree)

1. an amalgam of hungry and angry

2. when you haven't eaten in so long your hunger turns to anger and you say mean shit you have to apologize for later

Never feel hungry or have cravings again. Ever.

Warning: What it takes to keep yourself in a blissful world where you're never hungry and never have cravings for sweets can be really freaking hard. It requires two hard-to-come by, precious resources—time and planning. Great. The two things that no one has and likely the two reasons we have all failed at weight loss before. A magical world free from cravings does exist but what it takes to get there (time and planning) will be a hurdle you'll have to decide is worth overcoming. The question is, *are you worth putting that extra effort into?* Of course you're worth it, and anyone who truly cares about your happiness will support you along your journey to be the best *you* that you can be.

The way to never feel hungry or have cravings for sweets is to understand how to keep your blood sugar levels steady all day—never too high, never too low. You must find and stay in this Goldilocks zone all day, every day if cravings for sugar and constant hunger are what is holding you back from losing weight. Having a steady blood sugar level without peaks and valleys is the key to not feeling hungry. Write that down.

Steady blood sugar = not hungry.

Low blood sugar = hangry.

High blood sugar = wired, tired, then way too fucking hungry to eat sensible ever again.

So how do you keep your blood sugar steady all day so you never feel hungry?

1. Don't eat too much sugar.

Start reading all ingredient labels. If sugar is in the first few ingredients, set it back. If you must have it, then use these guidelines:

Eat no more than 24g of sugar per day for women.

Eat no more than 36g of sugar per day for men.

These are not arbitrary numbers I picked from bingo balls. Go to the American Heart Association's website if you want to read more about how deleterious sugar is for you and why to keep it within those guidelines. It can be found at www.heart.org

Sugar is the devil I believe in, and his temptations are real. Since the majority of us are sugar sinners, having a solid boundary as listed above can be helpful. Since no amount of added sugar is considered good for you, any amount over zero is not recommended. Total killjoy, I know.

Save your sugar grams and only eat the sinfully sweet things you *really* like while also staying within those limits. If you want to lose weight, reducing added sugar to less than the grams above can be enormously helpful. If there is one thing to try with all your might for weight loss, this is it.

If you were working with me and your number one goal was weight loss, one of the key things I would stick you to is not going over the allotted grams of sugar per day. Which is actually quite generous since if you ate 25g of sugar a day for 365 days you'd be consuming little over 46 cups a year or 2,282 sugar cubes or about 20 pounds— the weight of a small child. 25g a day is a generous recommendation. Sprinkle it here, sprinkle it there, sprinkle it anywhere you like, but Don't. Go. Over. Use your grams wisely, and no, you can't save them up for a few days and combine them into one item; these are not negotiable work breaks to be spliced together so you can go to the dentist. If you don't use them in one day, you lose them, and they don't carry over like your sick leave.

Like zombies and vampires in young adult books, sugar is lurking everywhere. It is continually trying to lure you, suck you into its blissful world, then steal your youth. You'll have to look for it in everything and *READ ALL LABELS*.

Don't. Go. Over.

You do not have to count fruit sugar *unless* it's from a can, a sealed plastic cup, or it's dried or pasteurized juice. If you have diabetes, you have to count everything. For the rest of us, in these forms, sugar is so easily assimilated into your blood that you have to count it toward your daily sugar grams if you want to lose weight.

Eat all the fresh or frozen fruit you want. If you

start counting grams of sugar in fresh fruit, you'll likely cut down on your servings and thus cut down on the disease preventing benefits these miraculous, colorful warriors are designed to give you. I do not believe cutting out fruit sugar is necessary or part of a healthy diet—period. Unless you have diabetes or suspect insulin resistance, eat all the fruit you want.

I will often hear individuals say "I don't eat bananas because they have too much sugar" or "I don't eat grapes, watermelon, or pineapple."

So I ask, "You don't eat grapes? So you don't drink wine then either. And I assume you've also cut out every last speck of added sugar from your diet before you cut fruit, right? Because why would you eliminate pineapple from your diet trying to cut sugar but you still eat chocolate or anything with flour or packaged or on the go."

To which they respond, "Well..."

Well, what?

Only if you have cut out every last speck of sugar from everything else you're stuffing past your lips and are still not losing weight should you even think about cutting out fresh or frozen fruit. If you are drinking alcohol or eating chocolate or any item with straight-up sugar, it makes no sense to put yourself on a weight loss plan that includes these indulgence items but cuts out one of the top two food groups that prevent disease and promote optimal health.

Cutting out sugar, or keeping it to less than the above recommended grams each day, will make a significant difference in your level of perceived hunger and cravings, not to mention the kick in the ass it will give your fat cells to give up their cache of blubbery goo. Eliminating sugar or keeping it under the guidelines is a *MUST* if you want to lose weight.

> "I just starting eating all this fruit
>
> and I gained a ton of weight!"
>
> —No one. Ever.

2. Eat plants.

Eating plants helps keep your blood sugar level all day—provided those plants still have intact fiber. Plants contain fiber, animals do not. Fiber fills you up and slows down the absorption of sugar into your bloodstream, preventing peaks. Eat plants, get fiber, curb hunger, go poop, repeat.

How much fiber? As much as you can; start slowly.

If you must have a guideline to follow, aim for 40g per day. Assume one serving (a handful) of fresh or frozen fruits or vegetables has 5g of fiber. That should make you poop your brains out pretty good.

3. Eat frequently.

Feed yourself a steady stream of energy throughout the day to keep your energy levels up and hunger at bay. Yes, I did intentionally rhyme that. If you go too long without eating, your blood sugar levels will drop and you'll feel hungry. If you let this continue, your body will wonder what the hell you're doing. She'll demand that you find an abundance of calories immediately or else she'll turn your metabolic fires down to protect you against the coming famine.

Let's say you've failed to eat frequently enough and your blood sugar has gotten way low. You wolf down convenience food or binge on sugar cause you're starving; now you've got a spike in blood sugar. Insulin comes rushing in to deal with all that sugar and its job is to pack sugar into your cells. When your cells can't fit anymore sugar in there, insulin will happily help to store the excess sugar as fat in your belly. Which will crash your blood sugar so you feel hungry again earlier than you would have if you would have just eaten at regular intervals. You get me?

Don't even give me that "I'm too busy to eat frequently" bullshit. So am I. Bring snacks. Leaving the house without snacks is like leaving without your pants. Be prepared with food in your purse, your car, your desk, keep some leftovers in the back of your mouth. In the winter, I throw my food on the seat; in the summer, I pack a small cooler. I usually have cashews, roasted edamame, dried fruit, rice cakes, peanut butter, packets of almond butter, and fresh fruit. I also keep convenience food like raw vegan snack bars.

Part II:
What

Chapter 9

"THE GREATENESS OF A NATION CAN BE JUDGED BY THE
WAY ITS ANIMALS ARE TREATED... I HOLD THAT,
THE MORE HELPLESS A CREATURE, THE MORE
ENTITLED IT IS TO PROTECTION BY MAN
FROM THE CRUELTY OF MAN."

—MAHATMA GANDHI

An argument for plants:

"The lower the percentage of animal-based foods that are consumed, the greater the health benefits—even when that percentage declines from 10 percent to 0 percent of calories. So it's not unreasonable to assume that the optimum percentage of animal-based products is zero," writes biochemist, T. Colin Campbell in his book *The China Study.*

I have so many highlighted, dog eared, scribbled on books with my favorite and heartbreaking passages concerning health, weight loss and the benefits of eating plants—I wanted to share them all with you, but my editor insisted it was a bad idea.

There are dozens of books that make a much more compelling argument against eating animals than this one. When I set out to write this book, my intention was not to tell you about the atrocities that happen inside slaughter houses or the havoc mass farming animals has on the environment. Although I would love to be overly dramatic here and persuasively argue my point for hours about why eating plants is a superior choice for all of mankind and this planet, I've decided to get in and get out. You can decide which issue to further examine; there is a mountain of evidence waiting for you on each of these issues.

Need a reason to stop eating animals and start eating more plants? Pick one:

- Pesticides are more concentrated in animal foods
- Antibiotic resistance from overuse in farm animals
- Methane and global warming from the mass production of food animals
- Animal food crops and the waste land they produce
- Depletion of ground water for food crops

and animal farming

- Confined animal feeding operations CAFO's
- Battery cages stuffed full with chickens
- VEAL
- Excess hormones used on livestock
- Eating meat and the increased risk of coronary artery disease and cancer
- Ocean dead zones from contaminated, fertilized farmland run-off water
- Algae blooms, fresh water lake die offs from contaminated, farmland run-off water
- The decimation of ocean fish populations
- The billions of pounds of farmed fish feces contaminating the ocean
- High levels of mercury in swordfish, shark, king mackerel, tilefish, tuna, shrimp, catfish, salmon
- Depletion of calcium in our bones from a diet high in animal foods
- Depletion of ground water and aquifers because we've used it all to grow feed crops for animals we consume
- Salmonella
- E. Coli
- Campylobacter

- Avian flu
- H1N1
- AIDS
- Ebola
- Creutzfeldt-Jakob (Bovine Spongiform Encephalopathy, aka Mad Cow)
- The negative environmental impact (drought, desertification) that traditional farming contributes to

Heterocyclic amines. It sounds like an STD but it's so much worse. Paraphrasing what *Cancer Survivor's Guide* explains, heterocyclic amines are cancer-causing chemicals formed every time meat is cooked. The hotter and more charred the meat, the more cancer-causing amines. Even "healthier" options like grilled chicken, when tested, contained the most amines.

Each of the above topics could occupy volumes, examining our folly and incredulous behavior. Making the switch to eating plants instead of animals was easy for me when the facts became clear. I could not, would not, contribute to such a catastrophic industry for myself, the animals, or our planet, any longer. I found the courage and resolve to come out from hiding behind this kind of dismissive self-talk.

"I'm too sensitive."

"I don't want to know."

"I love animals."

"If I know then I'll never be able to eat meat again."

"I can't bear to think about it, so don't tell me.

I used these excuses and others to justify my gluttonous behavior of eating meat. But these are no excuses. Ignorance is not bliss; ignorance is ignorance. If you love animals and care about the treatment of all sentient creatures on earth; if you don't want to participate in the unspeakable cruelty they endure so that you can eat them; then you only have to do one simple thing. Stop buying them.

Jane Goodall writes in *Harvest for Hope: A Guide to Mindful Eating*, "I recognize that for many people, giving up meat would be extremely hard. But if everyone knew and faced up to all the facts, most would either opt for drastically cutting their meat consumption and eating only free-range animals, or giving up meat all altogether. For the mass production of meat on intensive farms is taking its toll not only, as we have seen, on the well-being of the animal victims but also on human health. And it is wreaking havoc on the environment whether the animals are factory farmed or grazed."

I truly believe animals are not here for us to exploit and slaughter while plant food is in abundance. I'm not talking about hunting to feed your family; I'm talking about the mass production of animals as commodities in factory farms. If you can still live with yourself after you know the truth about what happens in order to stock every grocery store in America, I'd be concerned. As the saying goes, "If you're not part of the solution, you're part of the problem."

I could go on for days about why eating animals is fucking horrible for you and for the planet, most of it would be true, some would be embellished to get the point across. But in the end, the take-home message is that if you want to increase your life expectancy and decrease your risk of acquiring Western diseases, you'll make a slow (or fast) transition to a plant-based diet.

If you want to lose weight... well, the evidence is so undeniably clear. Plant eaters lose weight and keep it off. Period. Eating plants is healthy. Eating factory-farmed animals is supporting extreme cruelty.

...

All foods fall into one of two kingdoms.

Plants or animals.

It's that simple, eat plants. Make the ratio of plants to animals in your diet the best you possibly can. Strive for a 10:1 plants to animals ratio. Eat ten plants to every one animal food serving. A 10:1 plants to animals food day might look like this:

<u>Breakfast</u>

> 1 serving oatmeal with 1 serving almond milk, a handful of blueberries, a handful of slivered almonds
>
> *5 plant, 0 animal servings*

<u>Snack</u>

> Handful of grapes, handful of walnuts
>
> *2 plant, 0 animal servings*

<u>Lunch</u>

> Hummus, avocado, tomato, red onion and spinach on sprouted grain bread. Fresh fruit on the side
>
> *7 plant, 0 animal servings*

<u>Snack</u>

Hummus and nut crackers

2 plant, 0 animal servings

<u>Dinner</u>

Spinach and pesto quiche with chunky
tomato sauce

(A hearty portion would offer 3–4 servings
of vegetables with 2 serving of animal from
the eggs.)

4 plant, 2 animal servings

Daily total: 20:2 or 10:1.

A 5:1 plant to animal foods day might look something like
this:

<u>Breakfast</u>

Breakfast smoothie (Almond milk, coconut
water, 1 cup frozen fruit, handful fresh
spinach, 1/2 cup yogurt.)

5 plant, 1 animal servings

<u>Lunch</u>

Black bean vegetarian chili and cornbread, side salad with ranch.

(Let's say this totals 6 plant servings, 1 animal serving for the dressing and whatever eggs or dairy is in the cornbread.)

6 plant, 1 animal servings

Dinner

Pan-seared salmon with steamed asparagus and cauliflower mash. *(Note: a serving of salmon is roughly the size of a deck of cards, you'll likely eat more, probably about two servings worth)*

4 plants, 2 animal servings

Daily total: 15:3 or 5:1.

I'm not measuring specific ounces or serving sizes here; I'm only differentiating between plants and animals and assuming that generally one serving of whole real plants is one handful and one serving of animal is somewhat equivalent. Not science, art—food art. A little subjective, a tad creative.

Does this mean if you come over to my house I'm going to throw paint on your fur coat? No—because if you owned a fur coat we might not have enough in common for you to come over for dinner. But if you did come over for dinner in cotton clothing, I'll serve you the best vegetarian meal you've ever had; we'll drink wine and I'll play you a jolly tune on the piano in my kitchen, likely some obscure '80s song, and you just might sing along.

When you leave my house and you are still not a vegetarian, we will still be friends—because I like friends who are their own people with their own opinions which are inevitably different than mine. That's what makes things interesting and challenges us to grow, and think, and stay flexible.

Which would you rather? A friend who is a limp fish with an impotent handshake and no opinion? Or a friend with a backbone who will fight to get you back if you get kidnapped and taken to Mogadishu?

I want a friend who will still be a friend despite our differences and who would never give up if I got nabbed. So if that is you and you're still a meat eater, I can fall in love with you anyway. I suppose. But I certainly won't be kissing you.

WTF are you supposed to eat, you ask?

Plants.

Mostly plants.

Drink wine, eat plants.

Chapter 10

"FOR PERMANENT WEIGHT-LOSS SUCCESS,
YOU'LL NEED TO KEEP IT REAL."

Carbs.

20 percent? 10 percent? 100 grams? 50 grams? WTF, how many carbs am I supposed to eat? Since I'm not going to tell you a specific number of carbs in grams or percentage, if you want to "count carbs" then you'll have to figure it out on your own.

When it comes to carbs and weight loss, it's simple. You won't ever have to think about or count carbs if you eat a *mostly* plant-based diet of whole unprocessed foods. The more whole plant foods you eat, the less dense carbs you'll be consuming, and if you have weight to lose, it'll start coming off.

Like every other aspect of your food lifestyle, how you'll figure out what will work for you is by experimenting to see what works and what doesn't. Some of you might have to cut a lot because you eat a lot of processed flour crap foods and that's what your metabolism requires of you. Others will be able to keep endless pasta bowls on their menu and still stay skinny. Everyone's weight-loss plan should look different because everyone is different.

In the aforementioned book *The China Study,* T. Colin Campbell notes, "There is a mountain of scientific evidence to show that the healthiest diet you can possibly consume is a high-carbohydrate diet. It has been shown to reverse heart disease, reverse diabetes, prevent a plethora of chronic diseases, and yes, it has been shown many times to cause significant weight loss. But it's not as simple as that."

What he means when he says "it's not as simple as that," is that not all carbs are included in this statement— only a whole food, plant-based diet which is naturally high in what is frequently known as the "good" carbohydrates are recommended.

This is where you're probably expecting me to tell you to eat less starchy carbs and more protein. Or you're looking for a ratio of how much of what to eat. Like, (100g carbs a day, 60g of protein, and no more than 20g fat.) Maybe you're used to recommendations more like (your plate should be 40 percent carbohydrates, 40 percent protein, and 20 percent fat.)

But what are you going to do, fetch you're sixth grader's protractor and divide your plate into sections? Download an app so you can look up every single piece of food you put in your mouth then calculate how many calories of what is in it so you can map it out? That's not necessary if all you want is to be at a normal, healthy weight. If you want to look like a cover model, you'll have to track and map and get a coach and get your ass to the gym every day—more than once.

Do you have to eat a low-carb diet to lose weight? Of course you do, dummy. Low in the crappy carbohydrates, but not in the whole food, plant based carbohydrates. There isn't a brain on the planet that hasn't figured out that if the bulk of their diet is pasta, bread, crackers, cookies, pastries, and potatoes, their ass will be as wide as redneck double. Does that mean you should cut out all pasta, bread, crackers, etc., from your diet? It depends. How quickly do you want to lose weight?

I have two diets that work for me depending on what season it is. One is for weight loss. One is for weight maintenance. Both are healthy, one is stricter.

If we're going to Hawaii, I stop eating after 6 p.m. immediately when I know the tickets have been purchased. I won't eat bread, cereal, crackers, anything with flour, I'll stick to less than 20g of sugar, won't drink beer in the boat in the sun... boo! I'll juice a few days here and there, keep drinking wine, and I'll try to find time to walk or do yoga more days a week than not. In about 4–6 weeks—svelte. After we get back from Hawaii and it's - 40°F on our way home from the airport, I'll loosen how strict I am with myself—because I love food—not svelte.

I don't like being so strict when all I'm going to do is cover up under boyfriend sweats and a hoodie for the winter, and a little extra fluff doesn't adversely affect my health.

My off-season diet is a maintenance routine that will keep me within my Goldilocks zone but not on the light end. I won't lose weight, and I might slowly put those five to 10 pounds back on, but it'll take a few months at least. On my less strict food lifestyle, I drink what I want, order eggplant parmigiana instead of baking it at home the healthy way, and skip the gym to meet up for happy hour instead. I indulge in most social eating situations without much self-control. I actually like this life much better, but not when I have to be in a bikini. I like being skinny more than I like eggplant parmigiana. So inevitably, I have to be strict again at some point.

My bad food days aren't too terribly bad or I'd be a blimp. My maintenance diet is only slightly worse than my weight-loss diet, by American standards, even my worst days of undisciplined eating are still pretty clean. I eat 95 percent vegan more than not, but always a strict vegetarian. However, when you close this book and contemplate how to eat more plants than animals or give up eating animals altogether, you don't have to call yourself anything or tell anyone or explain or rationalize. You can eat WTF you want and never have to label it something.

If you need to drop weight quickly because you bought your wedding dress three sizes too small as an incentive, but now you've screwed off too much and only lost five pounds instead of 20 pounds, you'll have to do some pretty significant flour carb cutting. If you want to lose weight quickly, cut out all processed carbohydrates (anything not a whole food that grows in a garden) and all high-starch carbohydrates (corn, peas, parsnips, potatoes, pumpkin, squash, zucchini and yams) and all grains in any form.

Sounds drastic? Well, it is. But since you weren't

able to do something more gradually and now you have 15 pounds to take off in three weeks, this is what it will take, possibly more.

Eliminating processed flour-based carbs, starchy carbs and all grains from your diet, will drop your weight faster than the divorce diet. This includes sugar. If you have any hope of losing weight fast, the only sugar in your diet will come from fruit. Is it good to do something this drastic? If you need to drop weight quickly and don't give two shits about not keeping it off... yes, it works. Is it healthy? Depends on what you think fits within the definition of healthy.

Cutting carbs works to lose weight. But the drastic cuts above will not work for long term permanent weight loss unless you are 100 percent OK with never eating any of those foods ever again. Or if you're committed to doing hours of cardio each week to burn off the extra energy you're consuming before it gets stored as body fat. For permanent weight-loss success, you'll need to keep it real.

Be wary of the very low carbohydrate, one in which all fruit is out, no starchy vegetables, no grains, etc.... and basically all you can eat is chicken and more chicken. A diet low in carbs and high in protein slows down the brains production of serotonin. Serotonin makes you feel happy and *helps* to control your appetite. Low serotonin equals excessive appetite and cravings for carbohydrates. Enough carbohydrates in your diet equals enough serotonin to keep your appetite normal. So if you have no willpower like me, you'll need to keep your appetite and blood sugar under wraps all the time to prevent hanger and cravings and a potential binge.

Too many carbs will make you fat and give you all the related health risks that being fat includes. Period. But not all carbs are equally dangerous. Fruit, leafy vegetables, beans, lentils and a small amount of unprocessed, unfloured whole grains will not make you fat. Those are not the carbs you need to concern yourself with.

If you want to lose all the weight you could ever possibly want and be able to eat a shit ton of carbs every day, eat plants. Mostly vegetables, lots of fruit; a small amount of whole grains is probably OK for most people, and beans and lentils are a must. Since not all carbs are created equal, a high-carb diet of whole plant food carbs will actually work for weight loss. Not to mention what it'll do for your colon, kidneys, skin, energy, brain and ability to fight off disease.

Eat plants. Whole, real, plants are not high in the carbs that will pack weight on. So actually... I could recommend that you eat a very high carb diet for weight loss. But if I said that out loud too much or titled this book "High Carb Diet for Weight Loss" no one would buy it. Eat all the vegetables and fruits you could ever want to eat as long as they are in their natural state or very close to. Remember...

"I just starting eating all this fruit

and I gained a ton of weight!"

—No one. Ever.

...

I'd like to think that if I want to live the longest disease-free life I can, I'll have to follow what has been proven to produce that outcome. Well, tickle me muddy! It just so happens that there are populations of people who live long, disease-free lives.

I'm going to learn from them, copy them, study them, do what I can in my Americanized, highly-privileged life to imitate them. On my quest so far to imitate the healthy elders of the world, I've found myself eating a high-carbohydrate diet of plant foods for the last fourteen years and reaping the benefits of not having to worry about gaining weight beyond my healthy zone.

As the saying goes, "When you have your health, you wish for many things. When you lose your health, you only wish for one."

By today's mainstream standards, this is a high-carbohydrate diet:

Bagel and cream cheese, eggs, orange juice, pasta with veggies and chicken, raspberry iced tea, grilled chicken sandwich, baked potato, green beans, potato chips, and a brownie.

By today's mainstream standards, this is *also* a high carbohydrate diet:

Bowl of fresh fruit, oatmeal with walnuts and almond milk, black bean vegetarian soup and spring greens salad, sweet and sour tofu skewers with zucchini, peppers, onions, avocado and tofu with a side of curried quinoa, a brownie.

Example number one is the way in which we all have come to know carbs, so eating a lower carb diet would make sense if you're eating this way now. And if you are eating that way and you did cut those carbs, you would certainly lose some weight. If you switch from the high carb diet in example one to the high carb diet in example two, you would also lose weight.

So can you eat a high-carb diet and still lose weight? Yes. But you can't eat the typical American high-carb diet in example number one. To eat a high-carb diet and lose weight, you'll have to eat a whole food, plant-based diet.

Of course pizza crust is going to make you fat, of course whole wheat crackers and bread are going to make you fat—it doesn't matter if they are whole grain or not because they are still too high in dense energy calories for everyone normal.

Of course pretzels, snacks, chips, pop, anything with added sugar and anything with flour will make you fat—use your brain. If it's whole, real, plant food—eat it, even if eating those foods becomes a high-carbohydrate diet, you'll still lose weight.

One last point: if you cut out carbohydrates and replace them with proteins and fats, you're missing the whole point. Proteins and fats are good for you, no doubt, but should *not* be the bulk of your diet unless you want your spouse to pick out your cemetery plot unexpectedly early. Replace junk food carbohydrates with real food carbohydrates not extra proteins and fats. How do you do this? Eat plants, not chicken.

...

Here are a couple questions about carbohydrates that I hear often:

Are carbs really bad for me? What if I only eat complex carbs?

Carbohydrates turn into sugar (glucose) which you need to live, have energy, make babies, and run marathons. If you eat too much sugar and you don't use it all (if you haven't moved enough) then it'll get stored as fat. So if you are trying to lose weight and you eat too much sugar in the form of carbohydrates, yes, that's bad for your weight-loss program.

Here's the caveat:

Not all carbs are created equal, as you well know, because the word complex carbohydrate is tattooed on us at birth so we don't forget. Here's a reminder anyway: the more complex a carbohydrate is, generally the less sugar it has and the longer it takes for your body to turn it into glucose. This is a good thing. Eat carbs. But all carbs are sugar and will turn your ass into a cinnamon roll eventually if you eat too much. It's just that some will speed up the process more than others.

It's impossible to eat too many whole plant foods and gain weight. I suspect your jaw would tire or you would burn an equal number of calories chewing and digesting those plants that it would be a wash.

What are good snacks for low carb diets?

Anything that does not have a label or coupon. Now I'm just being an asshole, I know. Because that would cover 90 percent of the grocery store. To be fair, there are a few things in packages that'll work for limiting high-energy carbs, but not many. If you are eating low carb, I am presuming you'll keep to less than 30g of sugar a day (not including fruit) and are wanting something quick because if you had time, you'd have already roasted chick peas and cut watermelon to take with you, right?

So what can you get at the convenience

store that is low carb, plant-based and still OK for weight loss? Water. But you could also get nuts, oranges, bananas, or perhaps cheese. If you can get to a Whole Foods type of grocery store instead of the local Pack 'N' Pump, then there are lots of unique choices like kale chips, roasted soy nuts, quinoa crackers that'll fit in a weight-loss diet of high-carb plant foods. If you're daring enough to try them, and you'll have to be if you want options, most are quite good. The bottom line is that if you want to lose weight and cut carbs to do it, eating anything out of a package or a box is iffy.

Just so we're clear... if you're going to continue to eat junk carbs, you should go on a low carb diet of those junk carbs. Or you could switch to whole food plant carbs and eat a high-carb diet and lose weight. You pick.

Chapter 11

"INCLUDING FAT IN YOUR DIET IS NOT SOMETHING
YOU SHOULD THINK ABOUT TOO MUCH.
YOU DON'T NEED TO GO OUT TO LUNCH AND THINK,
'I'M GOING TO HAVE A SANDWICH,
NOW HOW AM I GOING TO GET MY FAT?'"

Eating fat might not make you fat—but it might give you heart disease. Are fats really that healthy?

The book *Cancer Survivor's Guide* points to the research: "High-fat, low-fiber foods boost the hormones that promote cancer. Specifically, diets rich in meat, dairy products, fried foods, and even vegetable oils cause a woman's body to make more estrogen. Similar findings have emerged about prostate cancer. Men on more health-promoting diets—that is, diets rich in vegetables, fruits and other low-fat foods from plant sources—are less likely to develop cancer in the first place and, if cancer does strike, are more likely to survive."

Eating too much of any fat, plant or animal, "healthy" or hydrogenated, is not a good idea.

The resource website Physicians Committee for Responsible Medicine notes, "Although the total amount of fat one eats is of concern, there is evidence that animal fat is much more harmful than vegetable fat. One study noted a 200 percent increase in breast cancer among those who consume beef or pork five to six times per week. Dr. Sheila Bingham, a prominent cancer researcher from the University of Cambridge, notes that meat is more closely associated with colon cancer than any other factor (Bingham 1988)." "Meat and milk are also linked to both prostate and ovarian cancers (International comparisons of mortality rates for cancer of the breast, ovary, prostate, and colon, and per capita food consumption 1986)."

The question is how much is too much? Research suggests that even small amounts. *Any* added oils while cooking, avocados, and yes, nuts and seeds—not to mention animal fat from cheese, milk, butter or meat— seem to increase our risk of coronary artery disease and many forms of cancer. Does this mean you can't eat coconut oil by the spoonful? That might be a bad idea.

"A close look at the cultures with low rates of breast cancer showed an obvious common denominator: a low intake of dietary fat and correspondingly low cholesterol levels. The same was true for cancers of the colon, prostate, and ovary, and for diabetes and obesity," writes Dr. Caldwell B. Esselstyn Jr. in his book *Prevent and Reverse Heart Disease: The Revolutionary, Scientifically Proven, Nutrition-Based Cure.*

The epidemic of low-carb diets has promoted replacing carbs with protein and fat as the desirable weight-loss alternative. For example, one recommendation might be instead of eating bread or pasta, double the chicken and add more olive oil into everything you eat. But this substitution is not the ideal; adding in meat, oil or dairy products in the place where whole plant foods should have been, is a bad idea for several reasons.

You'll be missing fiber, phytochemicals and antioxidants that only plant foods have, and putting protein in their place, perhaps because you think you need the extra protein which you may, if you're working out like a beast, or you may not, if you're just generally active.

Sure you might be eating a ton of protein and also eating vegetables, but what I'm saying is that if you don't need all that protein (if you're not a body builder) then putting even more plant foods in the chicken's place is the better choice instead of doubling the meat and adding oil.

Eating plants will keep your arteries clean. It appears that no matter what kind of fat or protein you include, the areas of the world that over-consume either, acquire western diseases. Whereas plant-based cultures that eat a minimal amount of fat and protein and exist on high-carbohydrate whole food diets do not.

Yes, some fat is good for you.

Yes, the Mediterranean diet promotes it, but that doesn't mean more is better. In comparison to the rural Chinese, the Mediterranean dieters have much higher rates of diet-related diseases.

Yes, fat keeps you full and helps level blood sugar but so does fiber. Decreasing your intake of all types of fats to a minimum seems to be the smart thing if you want to lower your risk of chronic disease. Now, I'm aware that in many instances, individuals increase their intake of fat and lose weight. I acknowledge that decreasing junk carbs and putting more fat into your diet can help significantly with blood sugar regulation and weight loss in some instances. However good it may be to decrease those junk carbs, replacing them with fat is never better than replacing them with whole plant foods, and it just might be reckless with serious adverse health effects *for some people.*

Some individuals can get away with eating more fat than others. Over-generalized recommendations like "eat less fat" or "eat more fat" are not accurate for everybody. Dietary fat and cholesterol does not always translate into blood cholesterol. Our cholesterol making process is much more complex than eat-fat = gain-cholesterol.

Every time I talk with a large group of people, someone always points out the person in their family who has consumed cream, butter, eggs and bacon every day since 1920 and is still living into their 90s and claiming good health or low cholesterol—by American standards. My tendency is usually not to believe them because for every one extraordinary claim like that, there are 10,000 more toe tags being issued from the very same diet. But this phenomenon does exist, in fact, this anomaly is in my family.

Great Grandma Rose has eaten her cereal every morning for 90 years with heavy whipping cream instead of milk, has consumed more sugar in her lifetime than grows in 100 cane fields, smoked Pall Malls for several decades, and probably never once considered *not* eating meat and potatoes for dinner.

Her cholesterol has always been and still is under

200mg/dL and her HDL's (the good kind that scrape your arteries clean) have always been within the considered healthy range in America. I didn't say she was healthy, but, in her 90s she has yet to die of heart disease or blocked arteries.

Her cholesterol may not be outstanding, but it's within the American "normal range." For most people, if they had eaten the way Great Grandma Rose has, they would have been pushing daises decades earlier. Great Grandma has beaten the odds.

Why her? Is a high fat diet loaded with animal foods and potatoes actually healthy for us? Did she keep her numbers within range from exercise or meditation? Bahahaha. No way. It's a rare genetic anomaly.

In Dr. Dean Ornish's *Program for Reversing Heart Disease*, he states that, "There is a genetic variability in how efficiently (or inefficiently) a person metabolizes dietary saturated fat and cholesterol. Some people can eat almost anything yet their blood cholesterol levels do not increase very much. (These are the people who sometimes live to be 100, and when interviewed attribute their longevity to the 12 eggs and sausage they have been eating for breakfast every morning.) Others find that even a small amount of dietary fat or cholesterol makes their blood cholesterol levels increase."

In a conversation with Great Grandma Rose about her diet, she is quick to point out her gluttonous dietary habits and the good fortune she has had with them—with a suggestive tone that maybe we all should be doing the same.

Enter Cousin Milfred.

I also have a family member on the exact opposite end of the spectrum. I'll call her Milf for short. Milf is in her forties, embodies her name, and has worked out (hard) every morning since the dawn of time. She is intelligent, highly educated, has three children and somehow still managed to maintain, I'd guess, no more than 15 percent body fat. For a woman in her forties, that's freaking lean. She's hot.

But Milf has a disconcerting secret you can't see on her beautiful exterior. No matter how much she exercises and eats healthy, to her dismay, she has outrageously high cholesterol. Over 300 mg/dL. The kind of cholesterol numbers you'd expect in someone about to have a heart attack; the kind that has to be medically treated so she doesn't kick the bucket while she's kicking someone's ass in kick-boxing.

Most of us are not on either end of the spectrum with Great Grandma Rose or Cousin Milf. The majority of people fall somewhere in between. That means, you might be on the easy end of the spectrum where you can get away with eating more fat and it affects your arteries less. Or, you might be on the difficult end of the spectrum where anything you eat seems to affect your cholesterol numbers, clog your arteries and decrease your life expectancy.

Since we can't change where we land on this slippery spectrum because it is determined by our genetics, we will have to accept the skis we've been given and proceed with caution accordingly. Start by figuring out how your diet to-date has affected your internal arteries. Go get your cholesterol numbers checked and figure out where you are on the spectrum.

"...if you follow a plant-based nutrition program to reduce your total cholesterol level to below 150mg/dL and the LDL level to less than 80mg/dL, you cannot deposit fat and cholesterol into your coronary arteries. Period." (Esselstyn 2007)

There, go write those numbers down.

Now you have a measurable goal that can be

changed with your diet. If you've adhered and it's still not enough, if you're rare like Milf (not likely), there is still help for you—statins. If there is anything in this book that might extend your life, it's this. Remember those numbers and do whatever it takes to get there because it *will* save your life.

I am somewhere on the easy end of the spectrum. I can still eat eggs, lots of them if I want, always with the yolk, avocados and nuts. I use oil in cooking when I want to, have a fatty binge or cheat meal here and there and still stay under 150mg/dL with my LDL's where they need to be—consistently well under 80mg/dL. With that, do *I* need to change the fat in my diet to prevent heart disease? I don't think so, if the above statement is true. Then I've found my Goldilocks zone on this issue and happen to have more leeway than most. My numbers look good, so I'll keep using that as an indicator of my internal artery health. But, if the day comes when my numbers change, I'll make changes too. I love my life too much to do anything stupid and jeopardize it.

However, we must also consider that dietary fat is clearly linked to breast and other cancers, so in that regard, I do my best to keep my fat intake to a minimum regardless of how much I can get away with and keep my cholesterol in range. This is part of my personal criteria to let me know I'm on track. Rather than assigning an arbitrary number of grams of fat that is recommended for everyone; it makes more sense to measure how much of what you should eat by the health of your arteries, your blood pressure, your weight and other factors in your unique biology.

Look at it this way, including fat in your diet is not something you should have to think about too much. You don't need to go out to lunch and think, "I'm going to have a sandwich, now how am I going to get my fat?" Just have a freaking sandwich—hummus, avocado, lettuce, sprouts, spinach, red peppers, add cheese if you must. If you're eating *mostly* plants, don't worry about where you'll get fat, it's in there. A plant-based diet will supply you with plenty of fat from avocados, olive oil, nuts and seeds (flax, sesame, chia, sunflower, pumpkin, almonds, cashews, brazil nuts, walnuts, pecans, macadamia nuts, peanuts) coconut oil, omega-3 fatty acids from seaweed or green leafy veggies, beans, soymilk, tofu, olives. You see? It's easy, so don't go freaking nuts here. Be sensible when eating fat.

Where you should worry about getting your fat is when you order something like a BLT and get way more than you need. If you want to lose weight, decrease your cholesterol, and decrease your risk of certain chronic diseases associated with the American diet; stop eating animal foods and start eating plants.

Chapter 12

"EVERY TIME YOU CATCH YOURSELF CHECKING
TO SEE HOW MUCH PROTEIN YOU'RE GETTING FROM
A PARTICULAR FOOD, IF YOU'RE READING A LABEL,
OR EATING ANIMALS, YOU CAN ASSUME IT'S TOO MUCH."

Oh, you're a body builder? I didn't know—you don't look like one. Do you lift heavy weights at least five times a week, rotating through different muscle groups in addition to doing cardio, stretching, and incorporating rest days as necessary to get ready for your next fitness or figure competition? If yes, then eating gobs of protein is what you'll need to do to get you there. But if the above does not describe your personal workout routine then you shouldn't be eating gobs of protein.

Eating a Herculean amount of protein will give you big muscles, yes, but only if you do the hard physical work to build those muscles. You also have to have the proper combination of hormones to support muscle growth. Eating an abundance of protein won't give you extra muscle mass or keep you lean if you are eating a whole lot of other shit too or not working out to build that muscle.

Protein *will* help to stabilize your blood sugar and kill cravings but too much protein might kill you. *WTF should we be eating?* Not more animal protein. The only population that need concern itself with not getting enough protein is... um... never mind there is none—at least not in any modern nation that has dollar menus and animal factory farms. Meat eaters get too much; whole food vegetarians and vegans get plenty.

High-protein diets raise homocysteine levels, which come with an increased risk of dying from coronary artery disease or from a stroke. This is a fact Dr. Caldwell B. Esselstyn Jr. (Dr. Sprouts) notes in *Prevent and Reverse Heart Disease: The Revolutionary, Scientifically Proven, Nutrition-Based Cure*: "A high level of homocysteine is very strongly linked with depression, schizophrenia, memory decline, and Alzheimer's disease... having a high homocysteine level doubles a person's risk for developing Alzheimer's disease while 52 percent of depressed people have high homocysteine."

Thanks to Dr. Sprouts and his insistence on a plant-based diet to prevent and reverse coronary artery disease, President Bill Clinton is still with us today.

Thanks, Bill, for admitting to the world that you're a plant eater and making it OK for the rest of us to come out of the closet. Check out the short interview about Bill Clinton's journey from McDonalds to a plant-based diet on YouTube—search Bill Clinton-Wolf Blitzer Weight Loss.

Plants have protein. But who cares? Stop thinking about how much protein you should get. We don't actually need as much as we've been lead to believe from popular media and big industry trying to sell you food packed with manufactured proteins.

Because I am concerned that you won't be satisfied at the outset of this book if I do not tell you how many grams of protein you should be eating, I feel I have to piss into the wind on this one. Wait... how can I tell you how many grams of protein to eat without knowing you? Without taking into account your activity level and whether or not the intensity you're working out at would require additional protein above adequate intake for optimal health? And all the other unique factors such as your age, weight, height, recent injuries or surgeries, medical history, chronic conditions, familial genetics etc.... I can't wholeheartedly give you a recommendation of grams of protein without knowing more about you. So I guess you'll have to remain unsatisfied on this, if that is what you were hoping to get.

However, I will give you this...

"Relative to total calorie intake, only 5-6% dietary protein is required to replace the protein regularly excreted by the body (as amino acids). About 9–10% protein, however, is the amount that has been recommended for the past fifty years to be assured that most people at least get their 5–6% "requirement." This 9–10% recommendation is equivalent to the well-known recommended daily allowance, or RDA. Almost all Americans exceed this 9–10% recommendation; we consume protein within the range of about 11–21%, with an average of about 15–16%." (Campbell and Campbell 2005)

And this...

"In some countries, the estimate [recommended protein intake] is as low as 2.5 percent of total calorie intake. The World Health Organization estimates that we need 4.5 percent of total calories from protein, while the U.S. National Research Council adds a safety margin and regards 8 percent as adequate...The World Health Organization builds in a safety margin and recommends around 10 percent to total calories from protein, or about

35 grams of protein a day. The estimated average daily requirement, according to the UK Department of Health, is 36g for women, 44 grams for men." (Holford 2006)

Lastly, this:

"0.5–0.7 grams of protein per pound of body weight." Which I clipped from the top hit of a Google search when I typed in "how much protein should I be eating per day?"

One more thing to make sure you are fully confused before I give you a solid answer on WTF to do. I've spent years in and out of different workout facilities ranging from exclusive all women's clubs to college university's fitness centers to strip mall joints open 24 hours. The protein recommendations don't deviate much from place to place in the fitness world: 0.7–2.0 grams of protein per pound of body weight.

So today I weigh 120 pounds, I'm 5 feet and 4.5 inches (thanks to the surgeon who gave me an extra half inch of height which stretched all my ligaments tight like a drum so now I can't even clip my own toenails). Based on the above recommendations, I need anywhere from 35–240 grams of protein.

Thanks. That's so helpful.

Like the quick lube place I took my car to last month for a quick oil change but instead I walked out with an estimate of $412 to fix some exhaust problem I didn't know I had. When I went to get a second opinion on my invisible problem, the other guy fixed it on the spot and charged me for 30 minutes of labor, or $35.

WTF is going on here? I'll tell you. Madness—pure madness. We've all gone bonkers with protein—jumped on the freight train hauling chocolate whey protein powder on its way to GNC and now it's so heavy and out of control it'll have to run into a mountainside of Granite to stop it, killing some of the unsuspecting passengers on board.

So how much protein should you eat if you're an average Joe Blow. Use this... every time you catch yourself checking to see how much protein you're getting from a particular food, if you're reading a label, looking it up, or eating animals or their byproducts, you can assume it's too much. Epidemiologic studies suggest we actually need very little for optimal health.

Should you ask someone for advice about your diet and the first thing they tell you is that you should eat more protein... move along. If you're willing to dig for the truth, it's out there.

"...animal protein consumption was associated with taller and heavier people, but was also associated with higher levels of total and bad cholesterol. Furthermore, body weight, associated with animal protein intake, was associated with more cancer and more coronary heart disease. It seems that being bigger, and presumably better, comes with very high costs. " (Campbell and Campbell 2005)

Eating too much protein, especially animal protein is not healthy no matter who you are. Eat plants, they will make you skinny and may just save your life.

Should I be drinking protein shakes?

Are you a body builder?

Do you lift heavy weights four or more times a week?

Are you an ultra-strict vegan or vegetarian who needs convenience protein to keep from looking emaciated?

Are you an athlete vigorously working out 10 or more hours a week or training for a marathon?

Do you have third degree burns over 80 percent of your body and require a feeding tube?

If not, you don't need to be supplementing protein with powdered shakes. Even for the special populations listed above with adequate knowledge and preparation, powered supplemental protein is not necessary. It's convenient—easier to drink protein than to eat a dozen egg whites, four chicken breasts and two cans of tuna, for breakfast (which isn't a good idea anyway). Protein shakes are a convenient alternative and do have a place in the world to produce a desired physique, just not with the general population for optimal health since generally on a meat-eating diet you get much more than you actually need anyway.

Ideal weight and having the lowest risk of chronic disease comes not from supplemental nutrition but from whole, real food.

Chapter 13

"ALL HUNGER EVENTUALLY SUBSIDES."

A few years back I was doing a one-day juice fast. I had my juice beside me in a glass jar when someone asked what it was. I told them it was fresh juice then elaborated that it was all I was going to eat/drink for the day.

She huffed, "Well... that can't be good for you—to not eat."

I replied, "What did you have for breakfast today?"

Begrudgingly, she responded, "I had cereal."

"Let me tell you what I've had so far today," I said. "For breakfast I had two tomatoes, two cucumbers, one head of romaine lettuce, one red bell pepper, a small hunk of garlic, a small hunk of onion and a teaspoon of red wine vinegar." I went on, glancing down at my muddy orangeish mason jar of juice, "For lunch I had two apples, four carrots, one bag of fresh cranberries, a bag of spinach, kale, and a lemon. For dinner I plan on having mostly greens."

You see, you could not eat all of those things in one day—but you could juice them. Then drink the juice and reap the benefits these life-sustaining, disease-preventing foods have to offer.

Should you juice?

Yes!

Unless you're diabetic, have high blood sugar already, or if you suspect you might be insulin resistant. In that case, get your shit together, change your diet first, and then you can juice when your blood sugar is within a normal range. Juice has a lot of sugar (fruit sugar) and when you're juicing and not eating food, you'll be damn thankful for those sugars that keep your brain working and your legs moving.

In a normal person, the benefits of juicing far outweigh any temporary spikes in blood sugar. If you suspect you have high blood sugar levels, you can still juice, you will just want to use greens and very little, if any, fruits.

"I believe that fasting is the 'missing link' in the Western diet. Most people overeat, eat too often, and eat a high-protein, high-fat, acid-congesting diet more consistently than is necessary." says Elson M. Haas, M.D. in *The Detox Diet.*

When eager clients come to me and want to lose weight quick by doing some sort of detox, I usually decline to help them in that way in the short term. I first try to get them to lose weight through habit change before we do some juicing. Only after someone has established a new pattern of eating—habits that will allow them to lose weight slowly, permanently; only when they've proven to me they can do so with little guidance, then, I will walk them through a juice fast.

Approaching juice fasting in this way makes it a very effective tool for long term weight loss. You can lose weight by changing your habits, but often times, the weight does come off slow, so using juice fasting to knock out five or 10 pounds can be a really great way to get weight off more quickly. In the long term, that weight only stays off if that individual goes back to their new established eating habits that helped them lose weight slowly before.

When someone uses a juice fast or another liquid diet to drop weight but does not do the foundational groundwork to change their habits and lose weight slowly first, whatever weight was lost from fasting will come right back on. Use juicing for its health benefits, and use juicing for weight loss once you have begun to lose weight already with your new lifestyle. When I do a juice fast, it's for multiple reasons, mostly to skyrocket my energy levels, boost my immune system and shed a few gluttonous pounds of fat that have crept on and are now bulging from my jeans.

This is what I do. A simple routine, not too strict—I find it doable. If it's too strict or for too long, I have a tendency to cave and binge and drink wine until I'm drunk and feel like a total loser for quitting.

Prep Days 1–2

Eat a clean, plant-based diet. I allow myself only one small serving of whole grains per day (my body seems to have zero problems with small amounts of whole grains or gluten) such as a small bowl of oatmeal, and one small serving of nuts. No flour foods, pasta or dairy. No meat or fish. No more than one egg per day (must eat the yolks too). I include all the fresh fruits and vegetables I want, and green tea (caffeinated so I don't get a headache).

Fasting Days 1–3

I have done 14 days on just fresh fruit and

149

vegetable juice. It was difficult, but not as difficult as giving birth naturally (which I don't recommend and still have PTSD from)—juicing is more of a psychological challenge than a physical one. But in the end, both are worth it.

14 days took some gearing up for. Doing 1–3 days is much easier to fit in to any lifestyle and to pull off. On the days that I fast, I have as much juice as I want, keeping it as green as possible. I sip frequently throughout the day to keep my blood sugar steady and I don't exercise. At all. Not even a walk. I've found that any exercise fuels my appetite and makes it nearly impossible for me to keep juicing and not dive head first into a cheese pizza.

I have to stay away from the kitchen, lock myself in the bedroom during dinner or go somewhere like the library where no one is eating or talking to me because on day one I can be very cranky and might just rip their head off and eat it with ketchup. Day one is hard but each day gets easier. For me, all hunger eventually subsides, and I never want to eat food again in my life I feel so outstanding, but it takes a handful of days to get there. Some people do fine on day one, some people commit verbal atrocities.

Post Juice Diet

Same diet as your prep days before fasting. Ease back into foods. Your stomach will have shrunk significantly, so eat small meals slowly or you'll feel sick.

If you are contemplating buying a juicer and making fresh juice (which is the only juice you can use for a juice fast, and the only juice you should ever drink anyway) a part of your lifestyle I'd recommend reading something more comprehensive like *Crazy Sexy Juice* by Kris Carr.

You'll want to get a quality juicer and have a book of recipes. Or, like me, lose your juicing virginity spontaneously. Be reckless; buy a juicer without a coupon at Bed Bath and Beyond, and fill your grocery cart with produce. Then go home, strip down to your bra and panties, turn on old music and stay in the kitchen until midnight getting acquainted. (Somewhere in a box there is actually a picture of me doing this.)

If you must wait for a 20 percent off coupon and read reviews before buying anything, consider also reading *The Detox Diet* by Elson M. Haas, M.D. which will offer many options, tips, suggestions and recipes related to fasting. If you have specific questions "like how often should I be pooping?" Or "how do I detox from alcohol or caffeine?" that book will cover it.

Chapter 14

Soy milk, almond milk, cashew milk, coconut milk, hemp milk, or rice milk?

WTF am I supposed to drink?

These "milks" are not intended to be used for just *drinking a glass of milk*. Infants drink milk, adults drink wine. No adult past the age of... um... *weaning* needs to drink their mother's milk, especially not humans suckling cow's milk. Milk is not necessary for continued growth or adequate nutrition after weaning.

The hormones in cow's milk that help a calf gain hundreds of pounds can help do the same for a human. I'm not even talking about *added* hormones; I'm talking about the natural hormonal composition of cow's milk which includes hormones to be passed along from mother to calf so that it can double in size. Today's milk is a convenience food we've become accustomed to using, not a nutritional necessity.

A choice passage from *The China Study* illustrates the problem with drinking milk:

"When humans drink cow's milk, it causes some worrisome biological changes in the body, one of which is a rise in the amount of insulin-like growth factor IGF-1 in the bloodstream. Researchers have known for many years that men and women with higher levels of IGF-1 in their blood are at higher risk for prostate and premenopausal breast cancer, respectively compared to those with lower levels... Large studies have shown that milk-drinking men have a higher risk of prostate cancer."

There's ample evidence of our intolerance to milk after the age of four when we lose the enzyme to digest it; a clear correlation between milk and its role in causing Type I diabetes; and a compelling explanation outlining milks inadequacy to prevent osteoporosis.

Milk may provide calcium that your bones could use yes, but only if you have enough Vitamin D to push that calcium into them. And only if you don't consume too many other foods or drinks like phosphoric acid, (found in pop) coffee or meat that make your body more acidic. Because if you do, now your body has to buffer all that acid—and the only way to do that is with... calcium, which is generally taken from your bones. This process of maintaining homeostasis will take precedence over all other goings-on, including any warning signal to leave calcium in your bones to prevent osteoporosis.

There are entire volumes written on each of these issues, and I've included resources in the recommendations section at the back of this book.

Most of us grew up using milk to cook and bake with, but luckily there are alternatives to sucking the teat. You don't *need* to drink milk, but if you are going to use it as a convenience food, here's some guidance.

Soy milk

Soy milk is sweet. It doesn't taste anything like cow's milk. It has a mild soy taste that in some brands is stronger than others. Use soy milk in place of cow's milk over cereal or in any recipe where a little sweetness is desirable. Even the unsweetened, plain, original soy milk versions are sweeter than other milk substitutes, so do not use soy milk in mac and cheese to nurse a hangover. It'll taste like you added a few spoonfuls of sugar to your salty sin. The dog won't even eat it that way. Because of its sweetness, soy milk does not taste good in savory dishes such as creamy soups or gravies.

Look for a brand of soy milk with limited ingredients. You don't need all that shit with added calcium or fortified synthetic something or other. Get your calcium from greens not supplements unless you want kidney stones. Keep it simple. Avoid added sugars. Buy the plain or unsweetened variety. Most commercially sold soy milks have similar ingredients. Some form of this is pretty common:

Organic Soymilk (Filtered Water, Organic Soybeans), Contains 2 percent or less of: Vitamin and Mineral Blend (Calcium Carbonate, Vitamin A Palmitate, Vitamin D2, Riboflavin [B2], Vitamin B12), Sea Salt, Natural Flavor, Gellan Gum.

Not exactly like eating soy beans off the stalk now is it? Is soy milk healthy? Probably not. Is it better than sucking a cow's teat? Hell yes. But just when you think the answer is becoming clear, reality whacks you on the side of the head reminding you that nothing is ever that simple—soy, too, has a dark side.

Do soy products cause cancer?

Should I use soy formula for my infant?

Will it make my son grow breasts?

I heard I should only use fermented soy products.

These are questions that are better debated in a longer, more boring book where a full prosecution and defense are required to sort out the ongoing debates. But good luck finding a book or resource that is so compelling with truth one way or the other, that you'll know the answer beyond all doubt. And don't send me what you find either—trying to convince me one way or another. I've read enough on soy that after every time I even think about the soy debate my brain gets frustrated and I have to do a head stand, take ten deep breaths and empty my mind so I don't attempt to drown myself from the spigot of my wine box.

I've raised all three of my kids on breastmilk, pumped both of my hooters around the kitchen table into the wee hours of dawn more times than I can count. When I couldn't take it anymore, when breast feeding and pumping no longer was *easy* or *natural* but made me want to scream in pain from mastitis, bleeding nipples and engorged breasts that could shoot milk clear across the room into my husband's ear while he was sitting on the couch, the time to stuff my deflated knockers back into a bra that I will never fill out again eventually comes. Then what?

If you can't breast feed your kids until they're six like the women from the pages of National Geographic, what do you do? The internet forbids you to feed your child soy formula, cow's milk formula or raw milk, in addition to anything non organic or not labeled GMO free. Oh, and by the way, steer clear of parabens, PEG, BPH, polyethylene glycol, coal tar, mineral oil, anything made from the back wax of a beetle, extracted from a sheep or emu.

It's all so fucking frustrating and confusing sometimes that when those babies of mine finally made their grand entrance, through what once was the tunnel of heaven turned into a screaming fiery hell, I closed the blinds, shut the doors, turned off my phone and computer and then did whatever the fuck I needed to do to survive— regardless of all the scary acronyms and plethora of opinions. I eventually gave them soy formula until they were ready to eat mashed foods. They drink water not cow's milk. My little boy does not have breasts.

Start where you are, make better choices from there, love your life, eliminate stress, and as they say in

Jamaica after you ask if there's seat belts in the car—don't worry yourself.

But regarding soy, I'll leave you with this.

A 2010 article from the journal *Frontiers in Neuroendocrinology* attempted to sort out the soy issue. Here's a snippet, "For a typical consumer, alarm over soy products is likely unnecessary but so is the belief that a soy-rich diet will alleviate all ills. Women who are pregnant, nursing, or attempting to become pregnant should use soy foods with caution and be aware that soy formula may not be the best option for their babies. Older individuals, especially those with high cholesterol, may experience modest benefits including improved bone and cardiovascular health, and perhaps a decreased risk of carcinogenesis. Moderation is likely key and the incorporation of real foods, as opposed to supplements or processed foods to which soy protein is added, is probably essential for maximizing health benefits." (Patisaul and Jefferson 2010)

Well, folks—there you have it. A little bit of everything, not too much of anything.

Almond milk

Almond milk is best used in savory dishes that soy

milk wrecks with its sweetness and potentially cancer-causing phytoestrogens (if they don't help to balance your hormones instead) but no one really knows for sure.

I've used almond milk in creamy cauliflower soup, mashed potatoes or cauliflower mash. In sauces that call for milk and butter, I substitute almond milk and maybe add olive or canola or coconut oil if necessary. But butter in recipes (not baking) is often not necessary to hold anything together; it's just added fat, just to add fat.

Leaving out the fat and using almond milk instead of cow's milk will not make the dish taste like the original, but the original dish might give you heart disease. Decide which you can live with. Play *would you rather?*

The ingredients in almond milk suffer the same set back as those in soymilk. They are as far from an almond as soy milk is to a soy bean:

Almond milk (Filtered Water, Almonds), Cane Sugar, Sea Salt, Natural Flavor, Artificial Flavor, Locust Bean Gum, Sunflower Lecithin, Gellan Gum. Calcium Carbonate, Vitamin E Acetate, Zinc Gluconate, Vitamin A Palmitate, Riboflavin (B2), Vitamin B12, Vitamin D2.

Luckily, almond milk is easy to make at home. In the recipes section, I've included an easy recipe for you to try.

Cashew milk

Same as almond milk. But generally, cashew milk is the best dairy substitute for cooking. It's creamy, dreamy, and delicious and can make the new dishes taste like the old dishes without the dairy. It can be used in pretty much anything and can also be made at home without added ingredients.

Rice milk

I generally avoid rice milk not because of its taste, but because it's high in quick releasing sugars (carbs). The extra carbs that I likely won't burn off and thus will only make me fat. For this reason alone, I avoid rice milk. I wish I didn't have to; I actually like rice milk, but like all the other off-limits foods for me, it sure would be great to eat them all without getting fat, but that is just not my reality.

Coconut and hemp milk

Suffer the same fate as the rest with lots of processing and added ingredients to maintain shelf life or sell the product to a bunch of unsuspecting consumers who think added calcium or vitamin D in everything you eat is a good idea.

Each of these milks have different nutrient properties with purported benefits that may or may not win a prize for promoting optimal health. But all of them are far superior than drinking cow's milk. Don't fall victim to the milk scam and get bent over the barrel by the dairy industry. Use nut milks when cooking, if you like, but you do not need to drink them.

...

Butter, olive oil, coconut oil?

WTF am I supposed to use?

Olive oil

Olive oil should not be used as your everyday cooking oil. It smokes when used even at a low temperature like 325°F. If it sizzles, pops or crackles, you shouldn't be cooking with olive oil. The only sound you should hear when using olive oil is the soft glug as you pour it from the glass jar.

Use it in salad dressings, over pasta, or for gluttonous bread dipping. Wait... don't pour oil over your pasta or dip bread in it if you want to get skinny. That will keep you fat. In fact, skip the pasta and bread all together.

Use olive oil with really low heat or none at all. One exception here; high quality extra virgin olive oil and extra light olive oil have a much higher smoke point. Both can tolerate a lot more heat. Better yet, use vegetable stock when cooking instead of oil at all. There are great recipes in *The Cancer Survivors Guide* that use all vegetable stock instead of oil when cooking.

Canola, sunflower, safflower and soybean oils

All can be used at a higher heat—425–500°F before they smoke. If oil smokes, throw it out and start over—next time stop drinking and pay better attention to what you're doing. Which one you use is up to you. We could discuss the purported benefits of polyunsaturated oils or monounsaturated oils and talk about "healthy fats" or discuss the implication of using too much soybean oil with its high rate of omega 6's which promote inflammation instead of omega 3's which will decrease inflammation, but that's all old hat. New hat is that adding oil, cooking with oil, worshiping "healthy fat" is *out*. Some is okay but if you eat a diet of *mostly* plants, you'll get it without having to add it in.

Coconut oil

Has the same tolerance to heat as butter—more than olive oil, less than canola, sunflower, safflower, and soybean.

It doesn't taste like coconuts. It's very satiating; you don't need much to feel like you might throw up from too much "richness." I use coconut oil in homemade versions of baked goods, as a substitute for butter in recipes that need a saturated fat to hold them together; and like a grandma, I keep a jar in my bathroom for my feet in the winter months.

My client whose name rhymes with Schmericka uses it every morning on her teeth to keep them white; my other friend whom I shall not name here uses it to give her husband a hand job—swears it's a million times less sticky than KY. I haven't taken coconut oil that far yet, but I wouldn't be opposed to trying. Although I'm not entirely convinced of its omnipotent powers.

Butter

You mean the back fat of animals? That yellow waxy substance that resembles the stuff inside clogged arteries? Of course you like the taste; it plugs into the same receptors in your brain as cheese and heroin. But once you get away from it for a few days or weeks, you won't crave it any longer. There are great substitutes, shop around and find one you like.

...

Raw or roasted nuts?

WTF kind should I buy?

Raw is best. Roasted is fine. Roasted nuts are not bad for you; rancid oxidized nuts are bad for you. It is possible that the roasted nuts you buy in the store are roasted at too high a temperature and the fats in them become oxidized. If you're concerned about it, you can minimize this chance by roasting raw nuts at home. Yeah, right—who the fuck has time for that? Well if you do, I've included a few recipes I make once every three years at Christmas when I decide to try giving affordable homemade gifts to my family and friends who have everything they could possibly need already. If you seriously don't have time to do it yourself and need roasted and salted nuts to survive, buy your nuts in a canister or in a bag that has not been exposed to the light.

Don't go fucking nuts on nuts though. A little is OK. A handful is a serving. If you open the canister and can't help but raid all the nuts, divide them up into baggies—1/4 cup servings or one handful. For me, I can generally eat all the nuts I want, not gain weight and my cholesterol numbers are unaffected, but I know not to overdo these so called "healthy fats." I'm just sayin' that for now, it doesn't seem to affect my insides adversely. I don't eat them every day regardless. I do have them when I like them—sometimes I like them in the tub, sometimes I like them in my car, but never do I go too far.

As for the kind of nuts you should eat? Well here we go again—should we eat Brazil nuts for their extra selenium? Walnuts for their omega 3's? Should we stay away from peanuts because they're more of a fungus than a nut? Fuck no. Eat nuts if you want to, but don't go berserk.

Eat a little of everything, (*mostly* plants) but not too much of anything.

...

Stevia, agave or turbinado sugar? Or am I supposed to use Splenda, Sweet'N Low or Equal.

WTF, is there any sugar I can use?

Stevia

Stevia is a green plant that is powdered or liquefied and is 300 times sweeter than table sugar. But it doesn't taste like table sugar; it tastes like stevia. There can be an aftertaste that does not go well in everything. I use it in oatmeal, smoothies, tofu pudding, lemonade and mostly I'm good with it—I like it just fine but others may not.

The processing of stevia into a usable commercial form is a little shady. It's difficult to uncover which brand of stevia is less processed and its sweetness not extracted by chemicals. The least processed form of stevia is for you to grow it in your windowsill and stuff it in your lemonade like mint in a Mojito. If you can't do that, then look for green stevia powder. This is the stevia that is not as sweet, since it is not an extract, rather it's the whole leaf dried, which is still 40 times sweeter than table sugar. You need much less of it to sweeten things with minimal to no impact on your blood sugar and zero calories. Sugar makes you fat. When you can use stevia or another less damaging sweetener, it'll help keep you skinny.

I have not used it in baking. I'm unsure about what happens to stevia when it's cooked at high temperatures and concerned that it may morph into some unknown chemical and turn me into a Martian.

Agave

Agave is the sweet nectar from the Agave plant which closely resembles the Aloe Vera plant. Each can produce a product with universal appeal—tequila and aloe Vera. I could drink agave from the bottle; I have drunk agave from the bottle. I've drunk tequila from the bottle, too, but I prefer agave (mostly.) Disclaimer: everything I'm going to say about agave might be biased because I just like it so much. I've even contemplated pouring it over my nude body to get the hubs to like it as much as I do.

It's incredibly sweet, and the most divine thing about agave is that it has no flavor other than sweet—not sweet with a hint of Anise or sweet with a bit of chemical aftertaste—it's just blissfully sweet, no more, no less. I use agave more than any other sweetener. That doesn't mean I use a ton of it, I just use it more than any other form of sweetener. I prefer its taste and texture above the rest.

Agave has a notorious low glycemic index which means 7 tablespoons of agave are the glycemic equivalent of 3 teaspoons of white sugar. However, agave still has carbohydrate calories that will need to be used or they will be stored as body fat. So best not drink it from the bottle, only use what you need. Agave *is* better than sugar for weight loss, specifically for someone who has insulin resistance, but too much of anything is just plain stupid.

Turbinado Sugar

Turbinado sugar (commonly sold under the brand name Sugar in the Raw) is white sugar with a little bit of molasses. It's basically brown sugar. In Turbinado sugar, the molasses has been extracted, making it white sugar, then some of the molasses has been put back, turning it brown again. Why? Who the fuck knows—it's still sugar, brown and white. It's a twist cone.

Sucralose, Equal, Sweet'N Low

Sucralose is sold under the brand name Splenda or Equal. Sweet'N Low is saccharin. Both are manufactured, not-found-in-nature sweeteners. Are they OK to use? You decide. Would you be willing to eat a peach that was not actually grown on a tree but was created by a mad scientist in a laboratory during a lightning storm? The lab peach tastes similar to the real tree ripe peach, but it does have an *off* taste about it, a tingle on your tongue that isn't there from a Georgia peach. Doctors and scientists say it's OK, but there are a few outliers that caution against it.

Are you OK eating the laboratory peach even if it has a different chemical composition than a real peach? If you're OK eating manufactured food-like products, then these are safe choices for you. If not, you'll have to use cane sugar or sugar beet sugar or something else that existed before you were born.

On the subject of manufactured food, when writing this book I was asked if I was going to talk about the pros and cons of GMO's (genetically modified organisms). I'm not. It's too long and hot of a debate for this book and I'm not interested in getting a barrage of activists at my doorstep. Both sides of the GMO debate have interesting points of which I have yet, maybe never, will choose a side to be on—although I would like to say that it never makes sense to diminish biodiversity of crops, animals and their habitats. Yet if we destroy our planet so severely that the only way to grow crops is by using GMO's, we'll all be thankful, but please, do we have to be so stupid as to push our planet to impending doom destroying all diversity in the process?

When this issue comes up I'm also reminded that we've been test dummies for decades. Whether it's food (remember Olestra that caused anal leakage?) or chemicals being released into our ecosystem. Remember

DDT and hexavalent chromium? Still today, as I reside in my house just hours from one of the largest oil fields in the U.S., I can almost hear the fracking. Perhaps the bigger issue here is that until it's not okay for us to be test subjects for big companies and their products considered GRAS (generally regarded as safe) according to the USDA now, and recalled later, GMO's and whatever else lies ahead will be fair game.

...

Quick oats, old-fashioned oats or steel cut?

WTF is best for me?

Quick Oats

Quick oats act like flour thus are turned into energy (sugar) much quicker than their natural state counterparts. Quick oats have been processed in such a way that reduces fiber and gives them a higher glycemic index. You want food that takes a long time for your body to process—releasing glucose to you in a slow, steady manner and keeping your blood sugar level even (thus keeping you not hungry and skinny). The fiber in oatmeal serves this cause unless it's diminished as is the case with quick oats.

Old-Fashioned Oats or Steel Cut

Both are fine. The difference is texture, cooking time, the way they are initially processed and their differing energy densities.

Steel-cut oats are the least processed and have the lowest glycemic load, making them the winners for weight loss. But nothing is ever that simple. I find that since a serving size of steel-cut oats is less than old-fashioned oats, eating less steel cut oats is more difficult. When I eat steel-cut oats, my tendency is to eat as much as a regular bowl of old-fashioned oats, but in doing so I'm getting almost twice the serving.

I prefer to eat a lot of food rather than a small quantity of super energy dense food—just my preference.

...

Flax or Chia?

WTF, do I really need to be eating seeds? I'm not a bird.

Yes, my little ducklings, these seeds, among others, have health benefits that are beneficial to both birds and humans. Seeds have different and unique compositions and thus wide variation in their nutrient profiles. When not overdone, seeds are a healthful appetite-quenching, blood sugar-regulating addition to your diet.

All of their specific and unique properties are too long and unentertaining to describe here. What you need to know is one recipe for each, so you can start to incorporate them if you have not already. I have included a few recipes with flax, chia, sesame and pomegranate seeds in the recipes section.

Seeds worth giving a try are pumpkin, sesame (tahini), sunflower, flax, chia, hemp, and pomegranate.

...

Whole Grain or Sprouted Grain?

WTF is sprouted grain?

Remember when your kindergartener came home with a bean in the middle of two wet paper towels in a plastic bag? The instructions were to keep it moist and set it on a window sill where it would get some sunshine, then check it in a few days.

Remember his or her excitement when a few days later you opened the musty paper towels to reveal the magical bean that had sprouted and now has green hair?

Or with a good imagination now resembles a single sperm?

That's a sprout.

Beans sprout.

Grains sprout.

And when they do, the nutrients in the bean, and its sprout, explode. Sprouts can be eaten plain or in salads, or dried then ground into flour. Sprouted grain flour is then made into sprouted grain bread.

Here's the deal: if you want to lose weight, flour products are not your friend, even if they are sprouted. So what if they offer a better nutritional punch, lower glycemic load and give you more fiber; it's still flour—and flour will make you fat. While sprouted grain breads are nutritionally superior to their highly processed cohort, if you continue to consume them in abundance, you will have problems losing weight.

I do eat sprouted grain bread. Sometimes with avocado, lime juice and red pepper flakes and sometimes with peanut butter and jelly. I don't generally eat a lot of other flour products so having this in my diet semi-regularly works for me.

...

Venison, Bison, Grass Fed, Hormone Free, Free Range

WTF, is there really a difference?

Of course there's a difference—in what those animals are fed, how they've lived, if they've been treated with hormones or antibiotics, the different nutrient composition when you eat them. They are like us; some of us have more intramuscular fat (marbling) than others and therefore would be considered a desirable meal, a tastier choice than someone who is extra lean, tough and chewy.

But is one a superior choice than the other? No. The superior choice is not eating animals or abstaining until they are raised and slaughtered humanely and only then, consuming a very small amount and nothing more.

I am of the mindset that if you're going to eat meat, go kill it yourself. Or at the very least, go visit it before it goes to slaughter so at least you know where it came from and if the "farm" it was on used hormones, corn fed them to fatten them up, or allowed them to graze the pasture for their short lives. Then find out about how that animal will be terminated. See if it's a humane and acceptable process for you. Don't eat or buy animals with a blindfold on.

In his 2006 book *The Omnivores Dilemma*, Michael Pollen takes a trip to the slaughter house. He states that, "Mistakes are inevitable on an assembly line that is slaughtering 400 head of cattle every hour. (McDonald's tolerates a five percent 'error rate.')"

The "error rate" he's referring to is when the cattle are not killed by the stun gun. Five percent of 500 cattle an hour is 25 an hour. Times an eight-hour work day equals 200, times 365 days a year equals 73,000 cows slaughtered with an acceptable error rate.

Because it's an assembly line moving at the speed of a walking escalator, after not being instantly killed there is no stopping the production line or profit would also be halted. The cow is immediately hooked—dead or not, strung up by one foot, kicking and trying to hold up its head up on the way to the bleed area. In the bleed area a cow would normally be unconscious but the "error cows" (200 per day) throats are cut regardless. They are left to suffocate and bleed out alive, apparently an acceptable atrocity in the food industry. I can only presume that one of the top three most horrible ways to die has to be getting your throat slit while you're still alive. I do believe that all sentient beings should be treated with dignity and humanity. The extreme cruelty error cows and all other food animals are forced to endure makes me ashamed to be within the same species that is able to do that to another species.

Put your food through this test. If you would not want your dog, cat or horse slaughtered for food in that way, don't buy it. If you don't know how your food spent its life and death, or what became of its remains, and you're willing to take that chance with your own beloved pet— then go ahead, buy it and eat it. But if you're not willing to roll the dice with a creature you care about; a creature that can feel the same pain and suffering as a food animal, then you can't buy it or eat it. In a society that has ample plant food available; food animals need not be slaughtered and raised in the unsustainable, atrocious way that is our current method of production.

The mass production and slaughter of cows, pigs, fowl, whales, dolphins, dogs or horses, I can only assume, is the product of extreme ignorance. Likewise, the exploitation of monkeys and chimpanzees for bush meat, sharks for their fins, rhino for their horns or lions for their heads is presumably the product of extreme poverty and desperation. If we all understood how the production, consumption and decimation of these animals was the source of so much strife, poor health and environmental chaos, we would have no choice but to choose to eat plants instead.

Be a responsible meat eater and discontinue consumption of unethically raised, inhumanely slaughtered or unsustainable production of animals that is not good for you, your kids or the planet. The science is clear about the devastating impact of raising animals for food on the environment and the health consequences of overconsumption. The weight of this evidence is undeniable.

· ...

Beer or Wine?

WTF can I drink and still lose weight?

Would you rather have six ounces of wine, or 12 ounces (one can) of beer? Both have the same Glycemic Load, (GL) 15. Which is considered to be a low-medium GL food. As opposed to six ounces of bottled grapefruit juice that has a GL of 75. A GL over 20 is considered high. So if we are only taking into account glycemic load, you'll have more luck losing weight by drinking beer than bottled grapefruit juice. Drink grapefruit juice, only if it's fresh, for the health benefits, otherwise bottled juices are out.

But again, it's never quite that simple. While

alcohol or beer in small doses does not have a high GL, it does however have calories that have to be burned or will be stored as fat. So perhaps the Franzia Bike Race my cousins partake in each year is not such a bad idea after all? I mean, why not race bikes, burn calories, while drinking wine from a box that's strapped to your back?

Alcoholic drinks with the lowest calorie content are the best choice for weight loss. Check out www.getdrunknotfat.com where you can compare alcohol calories. Remember to include anything you're mixing in that alcohol, which is probably more calories than the alcohol itself. I drink wine, or tequila.

You might want to try a shot of top shelf tequila. It'll only set you back about 65 calories and will get you exponentially drunk in comparison to one drink of something else. If you drink enough tequila, you might even burn off all the calories you consumed as you heave over the toilet. I don't always drink wine; when I don't, I drink tequila—the good stuff, not any of that bottom shelf shit with the gold label that requires salt and lime to get it down. Oh, and I've never tried the worm, nor will I ever. I'd rather lick the bottom of a teenager's converse sneaker. Well—maybe not I can't decide.

...

Fresh, Frozen, Dried, Canned?

WTF is the best?

Fresh is best.

Then frozen.

Then dried.

Then canned.

Dried fruits are a nutritionally good choice if you can burn off the abundance of quick sugar calories, but for weight loss, dried and canned fruit or vegetables and their juices are out. The heating process in canning destroys much of what was good in the food, including the fiber which acted as a buffer to slow down the absorption of sugar—remember? Try to get fresh or frozen fruits and vegetables whenever possible. Either are a good choice.

...

Brown Rice, Buckwheat, Quinoa, Soba?

WTF is with all these pastas?

If you want to lose weight eat none of them. When

you're ready to maintain your weight, have some, a little— a very little. Pasta is flour.

To minimize the impact of the pasta on your blood sugar, and thus how fast it can be turned into body fat, pick something with the highest fiber, lowest carb content. If you are eating these different pastas for the variety of nutrients then great, but keep in mind that pulverizing whole grains into flour can diminish much of what was good in it anyway. Everything that was in the whole raw food is never in its processed counterpart.

It is a shame that it takes all that oil and energy to strip our food down to its bare bones then manufacture synthetic vitamins and minerals to put back into it, when it was actually the best in its natural form. There is definitely something to be admired and taken from a raw food diet. I am not nearly ambitious enough to eat all raw although I respect the people who can.

...

Wheat crackers or nut crackers?

WTF is the difference?

Neither. Or—same as pasta. Pick something with the highest fiber, lowest carb content. Crackers are flour products regardless of their grain of origin.

It is worth noting that nut flour crackers generally are less carbohydrate dense than say... Wheat Thins or something similar. The base ingredient, nuts, by nature are lower in carbs than their wheat cracker competitor. Again, you're not on a low-carb diet, but these kinds of carbs will make you fat. A diet high in carbs that come from a whole food, plant-based diet will not.

...

Is Greek yogurt really better for me?

WTF, it tastes terrible, do I really have to eat it?

No you don't have to eat Greek yogurt. You don't have to eat any yogurt. If you need to re-populate your gut with bacteria, then you can get your probiotics from a different source.

Regular or "light" yogurt tends to be loaded with sugar or aspartame, which is fucking toxic. If not aspartame, then sucralose and if not sucralose, acesulfame K (don't ask).

Greek yogurt tends to have a lower added sugar content and much higher protein content, and if you still believe you need to eat a high-protein diet, go back and re-

read chapter 12. If you've been trying to lose weight and including yogurt without success, then it's time to re-evaluate what you think you know about dairy or protein, or anything. Try cutting out dairy and see what happens, you might get the surprise of your life—the weight loss you've been waiting for all along.

Chapter 15

Do you eat only organic?

I wish.

Did I mention I live in North Dakota? Fargo to be exact—you know, the place where we stuff dead bodies into wood-chippers. Eating all organic, all the time in Fargo is difficult. However, it is getting easier as more people move into town. Businesses are responding to the population boom and listening to their consumers demands. For me, eating local year-round is tough, too. Potatoes, onions and squash would be the only things available to eat November through May. That is, besides canned and dried foods.

Eating organic is always best—the quality of organic produce that has been grown in sustainable ways, on farmland that has not been stripped of its naturally occurring minerals from over-farming, is far superior than

183

a mass supplied grocery store orange. When you can, opt
for local, sustainable, certified organic or just small farm
not labeled organic foods. Who cares about the word
organic and its many meanings anyway—just buy food
that hasn't been sprayed with poison from the closest
place to your house. Which might be your own or your
neighbor's garden.

What supplements should I take?

If your friend sleeps with some dude she took
home from the bar then reports back that she had the best
orgasm of her life, if you slept with him, do you think you
would too? Maybe. There's a chance—but probably not.
There's also a chance she was drunk, feeling sexually
deprived, perceived him and the whole experience to be
more than it actually was because she was desperate,
lonely and craving results.

What works for one doesn't work for all. We
shouldn't be sleeping around with every recommendation
we hear just because someone else took it and it felt good
for them. That doesn't mean it will feel good for you. You
are not them. Your body needs to be cared for differently.

Ask yourself what you think you need and why? If
you're already taking supplements, then ask yourself if you

feel any different from them? Are they producing the intended results? Is it measurable? If so, measure it and evaluate.

If you are supposed to have more energy, do you? Rate it, track it, write it down.

If you're supposed to have younger-looking skin, do you? Take pictures. Keep a journal.

Don't take supplements on faith and just hope or assume they are working. If you need them and if they are quality stuff, you'll be able to measure or see or feel the intended results.

Remember that you only need what *you* need, not what is recommended on television at 3 a.m. Does everyone need to supplement vitamin D? Fuck no—not unless you want kidney stones, too. Can some people benefit from it? Absolutely. I am one of them—sometimes, in the winter, when I'm depleted, not before or after, and not all year-round.

When you are thinking about taking anything, look up the benefits, side effects, deficiency symptoms and research which kind is best. Do your homework. Read the label and find out what the "other ingredients" are. If you're okay eating the wax from the ass of a beetle or supplements encased in the boiled bones and cartilage of animals, go ahead, buy things blind without researching it first. But ask yourself this—would you stick some stranger's dick in your mouth without researching where it's been? No? Then get to know all about your supplements before even thinking about deep sixing them.

If you think you have vitamin deficiencies, the best "supplement" is juicing. Get a juicer. Juice the shit out of every piece of produce you can find and do it daily or as often as you can. Don't think about it as carbs, think about it as getting more vitamins and minerals than any supplement ever could give you. Think about it as getting healthy.

Whole, real food is not made up of vitamins and minerals, fiber and carbs—it's so much more complex than that and cannot be measured in a laboratory. You and food (*mostly* plants) grew up together over billions of years. You're not a natural carnivore; your intestines are 30 feet too long for eating animals to be good for you. Plants will sustain you, repair you and give you whatever increased quality of health you are lacking—more energy, less body fat, less cellulite, less disease.

Drink wine.

Eat plants. *Mostly* plants.

I do take some supplements, each for a very specific reason; each with measurable benefits. Currently, this is my daily routine, but it is subject to change and does change throughout the year. I go with the flow man, change with the seasons. I suggest you get to know your body and do the same.

- Liquid multi vitamin and mineral. I have used the same one for nearly two decades and have found nothing that compares. I gain no direct benefit or compensation from recommending it, it's called ProVitamin Complete.

- 500mg of Vitamin C

- B-100

- 100mg Alpha Lipoic Acid

- Powdered greens in a smoothie (most days)

I have used a lot of "greens" products in my life. Everything from Juice Plus to the crap sold on the end aisle of Wal-Mart. I have found no better product than the Greens Powder from the company It Works. I gain no direct benefit or compensation from recommending it. This is where I get it from: www.wraphappy.myitworks.com

I believe in the power of antioxidants. Because there are dozens of antioxidant supplements I could take, and I have, but I can't take them all, and I shouldn't; I've narrowed down what works for me via education, and experimentation. My antioxidant routine consists of a mostly whole food, plant-based diet loaded with colorful fruits and vegetables with an emphasis on fresh berries and the greenest of greens.

In addition, I've said before that I drink green tea every morning and red wine every evening—not by accident, by design. On top of that, Alpha Lipoic Acid (ALA) works topically for the skin, which I've seen and use firsthand, but also, even better, it works internally. How do I know ALA works? Because after a few months of not taking it I look old—der. I can see it in my face; I look less rested, dehydrated and seem to have more wrinkles—all cellular damage that can be mitigated by antioxidants such as ALA, Vitamin C, green tea, red wine and others... I can't even tell you how much I love antioxidants—almost as much as I love wine, sushi, and my husband—at the same time.

In my lifetime, for different reasons, I have taken a plethora of other supplements. I suppose a lot of that experimenting was *just to see* if they worked like they were purported to work. Some have. Some haven't. But that doesn't discount their validity, all it says is that whatever *it* was, didn't do anything for me. Perhaps I wasn't deficient in what I was taking.

I've scoured the shelves at the local supplement stores looking for herbs and tinctures that will keep me young and skinny. I've been sold snake oil that will eat away tumors and devour scar tissue. I've been duped, susceptible at times to a good salesman, but in the end I've figured out I don't need much to maintain good health, youthful skin, a sharp mind and a healthy libido—for me it's just a few extra antioxidants and some greens that turn my poop the color of grass.

You don't need an ocean of pills. Start with whole plant food, then juice, then supplement if you feel it necessary for the specific areas of concern.

Should I stay away from gluten?

Gluten is a protein found in some grains, most commonly wheat, barley and rye. Celiac disease is a serious autoimmune disease in which a person's body creates antibodies that attack the small intestine when gluten is ingested.

In other words—if you have Celiac disease, your body fucking hates gluten so much it would rather die than have to deal with it. Symptoms of Celiac vary from abdominal bloating and gas to chronic diarrhea or constipation. More severe symptoms could be anemia, depression and anxiety, osteoporosis, joint pain, headaches and there's plenty more. If you suspect you have Celiac go to your doctor right now.

If you don't, should you avoid gluten?

Maybe.

There is a simple little test to see if avoiding gluten will eliminate undesirable symptoms such as the inability to lose weight, bloating, gas, abdominal pain, headache etc....

Stop eating it.

Go do your research about gluten intolerance, Celiac, what to avoid, and what's OK to eat, and then put yourself on an elimination diet. Stop eating gluten for at least two weeks. Keep a journal along the way to document how you feel each day and what you've eaten.

Write down if you notice changes in energy, irritability, weight loss, and appetite. If you feel noticeably better after two weeks, you may have found the unicorn. If you don't feel noticeable changes then whatever amount of gluten you were consuming before probably isn't enough to cause problems.

It's still a good idea to eliminate or significantly reduce all grains, not necessarily just gluten, if you want to lose weight. But especially wheat, even if you're not gluten intolerant. We can develop an intolerance to foods we eat too often and wheat is a gigolo who whores around everywhere he can. It's not really his fault though; the onus falls on the pimps that put him in every product that will take him in. Wheat has found a way to stick his kernels in everything you eat whether you want him there or not.

How can I make tofu taste good?

Don't eat it. Bahahaha... Actually, that's not true, but whatever you do, don't take it out of the package and assume it's ready to eat. If you do, you'll never eat it again. If you've had tofu from a buffet, that is often how it is served—which is why a whole population has turned against it. Served from the box raw it has a blah flavor and watery jelly-like texture. To make tofu desirable and juicy, you have to give it a little bit of foreplay.

When you buy tofu there are two types. Silken (the little rectangular, tightly-sealed box) and regular (square plastic package with a brick of tofu in water). The difference that matters is their texture.

Use silken tofu in desserts, blender recipes or anything with a hand mixer.

Use regular tofu for everything else.

Silken tofu does not hold up well if you try to cut it or shape it. It's crumbly and... silky. Silken tofu can be used instead of cream cheese, mayonnaise, yogurt, pudding, ricotta, or anything with a creamy texture. Use regular tofu when cooking everything else.

If you want it to have a "meaty" texture, throw the package (not silken) in the freezer. After it's frozen, thaw it out in the refrigerator for 24 hours before you want to use it. When you take it out, it will feel like a sponge. Squeeze all the water out.

What's left will be tofu that has a dense, meaty texture—great to use in a savory dish. In this form, it will do well baked, pan fried or put into a chili or stir fry recipe. *But* it will still be bland, so you have to season or marinade it with whatever you're cooking it with.

Tofu will take on whatever flavor you want it to, or it will take on the flavor of what it's being cooked with. If you like teriyaki, use it. Sweet and sour, fine. Peanut sauce, great. Use whatever seasonings or sauces you like. I like herbs (basil, oregano, rosemary, thyme) with sea salt and black pepper. Curry also works well with tofu. I simply prepare it, season it, and bake it. Or I throw it in with any dish I want, and it assumes the flavor of the dish.

When working with it raw (right out of the package), press as much water out of it as you can. Cut it into steaks, and put it on a baking sheet with potatoes, cauliflower and broccoli. Then season everything with herbs, sea salt and pepper, bake it for 30 minutes at 350°F. It tastes great, the texture is not raw—it's a little crisp outside, softer inside. It works and it's quick.

Should I follow a low glycemic diet?

If you're diabetic, yes. Otherwise, not necessarily. BUT you might want to pay attention to it—especially if you carry the most of your weight in your belly whether you're an apple shape or not. Doing some further research into Glycemic Load (GL) and following a low GL diet, could help you get some weight off. Until then, here is a quick lesson in GL.

Every food has a glycemic index (GI), a number which measures how much impact that food has on your blood sugar. Glycemic load uses the glycemic index number in conjunction with a specific quantity of that food, which accounts for its amount of carbohydrate. Did I lose you?

This might be tricky to understand. So in other words—you can play the game *would you rather* with any of the equivalents below. All of these foods in *these quantities* have the same GL even though they might not have the same GI. So eating half of one cake doughnut affects your blood sugar the same as eating 1.5 servings of quinoa.

Of course quinoa is better for you than a cake doughnut in terms of nutrition but the GL of both foods illustrates that even foods that are good for you like quinoa, can affect your blood sugar pretty significantly, which can lead to body fat gain especially around your waist. If you have a problem with insulin resistance or diabetes, this matters. If you don't, it might not. But, for some, paying attention to GL will help them lose weight, especially in their belly. Why especially in the belly you ask? Let me tell you.

In her book *The Schwarzbein Principle*, Dr. Diana

Schwarzbein states that, "I call the fat deposition around the midsection the "insulin meter" because this is an area where insulin first deposits extra fat. When I see patients with an excess of body fat around their midsections, I immediately know they have an insulin imbalance."

Insulin is secreted by your pancreas in response to sugar in your blood. Insulin's job is to push that sugar into your cells to get it out of your blood and to keep your blood sugar balanced. Here's the problem: your cells are already full of sugar from a lifetime of eating like shit and consuming too much sugar in the form of carbohydrates like pasta or bread, or simple sugars like those in coffee creamer, yogurt, or lemonade.

When insulin comes knocking on the door to your cells, it's overflowing with sugar and begging your cells to share the load. Your cells then, rightfully so, give insulin the finger and pad lock every door to the house so he can't get in no matter what his special pleading is. In a last ditch effort to penetrate your house, the pancreas secretes more insulin. Now that insulin has multiplied itself, it's standing outside every door and window huffing and puffing and about to blow your shit in, therefore forcing its sugar upon you.

Now, like your cells, I have a plan in place in the

event someone or a bunch of someones are about to break into my house. First, my place is fucking jacked with a security system like an Irish castle clad with its own moat and dragon—fit with motion detectors, sensors on every window and possible entry point and an immediate dispatch to 911. Let that bitch come knocking, no one's pouring some sugar on me without the alarms sounding.

But, if the intruder calls for reinforcements and is now outside every window and door, as insulin does to your cells, like your cells, I have planned for that too. My plan may or may not look like the movie Home Alone and involve a face full of bear spray and tower of toddler bikes piled on top of a mini trampoline.

So they all turn tail and run (if they can still walk) but unlike insulin, I have no idea where they are going and don't care. But we do know where insulin goes after it is shut out by your reinforced fortress. Insulin is taking those sugar molecules out for a night on the town, turning them into fat and leaving them smack dab in the middle of your belly. That is insulin's job. When the cells say no, they divert sugar to fat storage—in your mid-section.

The only real way to protect our cells from intruders is to not invite them in by eating a diet low in sugar. Which can be measured by a low GL diet.

These are GL equivalents:

- 1/2 of a cake doughnut

- 1 slice of white bread

- 1/2 of a bagel

- 1 and 1/2 servings of quinoa (*keen-wah*)

- 1/2 serving of white rice

- 2 rice cakes

Glycemic load equivalents show just how damaging high sugar foods can be on your weight-loss program. Remember, if your blood sugar stays level, you won't feel hungry, and if you consume too much of any high glycemic (sugar loaded) food, you'll have to use all that energy you've consumed or you will store it as body fat.

Here are a few other comparisons. All of the items listed below are GL equivalents. Choose wisely. Play *would you rather?* Would you rather have two baskets of strawberries or four jelly beans? Because those quantities of those foods affect your blood sugar in the same way.

- 2 large baskets of blackberries

- 2 large baskets of raspberries

- 2 large baskets of strawberries

- 2 large pears

- 2 large slices of watermelon

- 20 grapes

- 8 plums

- 2 small apples

- 1 banana

- 20 raisins

- 2 dates

- 1 small stick of Twix

- 4 jelly beans

- Half of a Mars bar

- 1/2 cup of regular soda

- 4 large tubs of hummus

- 6 cups of soybeans

- 2 cups of lentils

- 1 and 1/2 cups chickpeas

- 1 very small serving of macaroni noodles

- 1 very small serving of rice noodles

- 1 very small serving of brown rice pasta

- 8 pretzels

- 5 bunches of asparagus

- 267 servings of pumpkin

- 10 avocados

- 1 small sweet potato

- Half of a baked potato

- 5 tomatoes

- 5 handfuls broccoli

- 10 handfuls kale

- 10 handfuls of green beans

- 2 carrots

- 5 tablespoons of peas

...

"If you have failed to lose weight on low-fat diets, insulin resistance may be your problem, in which case you want to moderate consumption of high-glycemic-index foods. People who develop insulin resistance usually have high serum triglycerides, gain weight easily, especially in the abdomen, and often crave carbohydrates," says Andrew Weil, M.D. in *8 Weeks to Optimum Health.*

What is the quickest way to lose five pounds?

Juice fast.

Eat a pre-juicing diet for two days as described in chapter 13. Fruits and veggies, nuts, no grains, no meat, no dairy, no salt, no shit. Then juice for three days. All fresh fruits and vegetables, all day, a little at a time. No solid foods or fiber or protein other than what's in the greens. No exercise. None.

Walk if you like, but don't go running or lifting weights during this time. Use it as a time of healing and rest for your body and your mind. You won't be taking in substantial protein calories so why go workout hard when you won't be able to refuel properly?

Can you do it? Yes. It's not as hard as you might think. *OK, it's a little hard.* But you asked to lose weight quickly, so what'd you expect—an easy quick fix? Bahahaha! Nothing about weight loss is that *easy*.

I need sweets! What can I do to satisfy my craving?

Don't buy sugar-free pudding or some low-calorie Skinny Cow shit. A low calorie substitute often does not satisfy the beast and thus you end up eating more of the substitute and might as well have just had what you really fucking wanted instead.

If you want to curb your sweet tooth, you have to put on a condom and practice prevention. Stop eating shit that spikes and drops your blood sugar so you won't be able to think coherently and all you do is crave sweets. If you are hungry, your blood sugar is low, and you will have little willpower to say no when quick sugar calories cross your path. So don't let yourself get into this situation. Don't get overly hungry—that is how you stop the sweets cravings.

Carry snacks with you at all times, so when you get to the grocery store on your way home from work, you don't buy all that spontaneous crap you see and binge on the drive home.

Pack food in your purse, in your car, at your desk, and be prepared at all times to eat a little healthy to keep your energy levels up and your blood sugar steady so you don't get cravings in the first place.

Let's say you failed and now you're dying to have something sweet. If you try to fend off the craving until 10 p.m. and then you cave, that's worse than if you would have just given in at 4 p.m.

Eat what you really like; give in to your cravings sooner rather than later if you must. But you must make a trade off. You can't have it all, all the time. On the buffet at the family reunion you will have to choose what you really want and give up something else. Pick it, lick it and stick with it. Now get the fuck away from the table and go find a game to play on the grass with the kids.

Are soy burgers or chicken substitutes OK?

Remember, you are not making changes for a competition to win a medal for who can eat the healthiest. You are making better choices than you have made in the past. You are starting where you are and moving one rung up at a time. Unless you are really sick, or really overweight and it is life threatening. Then you don't have time for small changes, you'll need to get your ass moving with radical changes to produce radical results.

But if your life is not in eminent danger, your choices can be a progression from bad-to-better, better-to-good, good-to-excellent. For the rest of your life you'll take two steps forward, one step back on a continuum that never ends. Start where you are, make better choices; this process never ends. Be the best you can be. Eat the healthiest you possibly can, strive to be better, but start where you are, not where someone else is.

By this measure, everyone will be starting at a different point on the continuum. So where one person might say "I'd never eat those soy patties. Don't you know they're highly processed and not that good for you?" another person's viewpoint might be "I know they aren't the greatest choice but they are a hell of a lot better than eating the meat burgers I used to."

Both are true.

The meat substitutes can assist in the transition from a meat-eating diet to a more plant-based diet. As you get more acquainted with eating plants, you can back off the patties and only use them for convenience.

However, there are some "substitutes" that are not processed at all and are great choices regardless of where you're at on the continuum. Those are the ones that contain whole, real ingredients like black beans, barley, bell peppers, etc.... and have little or no preservatives or are made in your kitchen. If you don't have the time to prepare homemade spicy black bean burgers, *some* store bought ones are an excellent option.

How healthy are those protein shake places?

It depends.

If what you usually do is scurry through the drive through at a fast food place and order anything other than a salad, then going to a protein shake place or smoothie bar is a better choice. At the very least you'll probably get a serving of fresh fruit and a fourth of the artery clogging fat you'd otherwise get from a fast food place. If your option is on-the-go fast food or a powdered protein mixed with fruit, then I'd opt for the lesser calorie, less harmful choice.

Are those places a good choice overall for optimal health? They are somewhere on the continuum. Nothing is better than eating real food, *mostly* plants. That is what is going to give you the lowest possible risk of disease and keep you skinny forever.

But are those places actually *bad* for you? It depends. They are not bad for you if you put them side by side with bar food. But don't use a powdered mix or liquid food meal replacement instead of whole, real plant food a majority of the time. Eating powder versus eating food will never be a more healthful choice, but there are definitely a lot worse things you could be putting in your body.

When it comes to non-food foods, read the ingredients of what you're consuming then think critically; you'll know what to do. If it is whole, real food dehydrated, frozen or dried and powdered, then it's not as great of quality as the fresh stuff, but it's better than an isolated form of food like "protein isolate" or an extract like "bromelain" (a mixture of enzymes found in pineapples that is known for its anti-inflammatory properties.)

Bromelain is excellent for you in its original unadulterated form—which is inside fresh pineapple. It's the stuff that makes your tongue tingle and your mouth feel slightly burned or swollen. Bromelain breaks down protein (your tongue) so ironically as you eat it, it is also eating you. But you don't get that with canned pineapple or supplemental bromelain. Why? Because the processing of fruit when canning and other methods of preserving fruit, destroys much of what was healthy about the fruit to begin with, including vitamin C and enzymes like... bromelain.

When buying non-food food all of it will be processed in some way, that's why it's non-food food. It's edible like food, but it doesn't naturally exist as food. At this point in our food science technology, manufactured food is less beneficial than the fresh real thing.

But some food-ish products are better than others. For example, this is the list of ingredients in a popular protein shake/meal replacement powder that is widely commercially available:

Fructose, Lecithin Powder, Soy Protein Isolate, Maltodextrin, Calcium Caseinate, Sodium Caseinate, Corn Bran, Flavors And Artificial Flavors, Guar Gum, Lecithin Liquid, Magnesium Oxide, Carrageenan, Disodium Phosphate, Citrus Pectin, Honey Powder, Silicon Dioxide, Ascorbic Acid, Ferrous Fumarate, Potassium Iodide, Dlalpha Tocopheryl Acetate, Sodium Selenite, Niacinamide, Copper Gluconate, Zinc Oxide, Manganese Sulfate, Biotin, Papain, Bromelain, Vitamin A Palmitate, D-Calcium Pantothenate, Pyridoxine Hydrochloride, Thiamine Mononitrate, Riboflavin, Folic Acid, Chromium Chloride And Sodium Molybdate.

This is the ingredient list from a lesser well known protein supplement/meal replacement used in the same manner as the product above

Pea Protein, Whole Flaxseed (Micro-Milled), Cocoa Powder, Organic Acacia Gum (Naturally Occurring Fiber), Hemp Protein, Saviseedtm (Sacha Inchi) Protein, Organic Gelatinized Maca Root, Organic Broccoli, Organic Spirulina, Organic Kale, Organic Marine Algae Calcium, Fruit And Vegetable Blend (Spinach, Broccoli, Carrot, Beet, Tomato, Apple, Cranberry, Orange, Blueberry And/Or Bilberry, Strawberry, Shiitake Mushroom), Chlorella Vulgaris (Cracked Whole Cell), Papaya Extract, Probiotics (Bacillus Coagulans [Provides 1 Billion Cfu/Serving]), Antioxidant Fruit Blend (Grape Seed Extract, Organic Pomegranate, Acai, Mangosteen, Organic Goji, Organic Maqui), Contains 2 Percent or Less of:, Beet Root Powder (For Color), Natural Chocolate Flavor, Natural Vanilla Flavor, Natural Caramel Flavor, Natural Hazelnut Flavor, Stevia Extract, Citric Acid.

Which would you rather?

It would take me sixteen pages to go through the differences between these, the ingredients, their origin, how they are processed, the claims, the warnings. If I have to explain why the second product is far superior, then you must have been dozing off the last hundred pages. Wake up, go back, and read it again. You can find the second product here. myvega.com

However, if you've felt I've tricked you with these

options, I did. You might have concluded that neither was a healthy choice since I flogged protein for a full chapter and a half. Why would I now be saying protein supplements are good? I didn't. I said some products are better than others but real food is always best and we don't need all that excess protein. However, here is where it might be more beneficial to have a quality product than to not have it.

My hubs supplements protein. I order it for him. The kind I prefer to buy is Vega. There are other suitable ones as well but the quality of ingredients in this particular brand is outstanding. My hubs is a vegetarian, works out four or more days a week, has the metabolism of a fourteen-year-old boy, forgets to eat during the day and will often eat breakfast then nothing until dinner at 6 p.m.

On a bad day, he does not consume enough calories, protein or otherwise, to meet his basal metabolic requirements let alone make any gains from his workouts. Good thing he has some good days mixed in. If he doesn't supplement something, not just protein, as a male vegetarian, mostly vegan, with his limited ability to eat enough food during the day, he'll wither and die. His lifestyle requires food to be convenient if he is going to eat during his day. In this scenario, he is much better off with a quality vegan well-rounded food supplement than without.

Pea protein, hemp protein, brown rice protein and flaxseeds are all good choices for protein supplements if needed. Whey is not my first pick nor is soy my first protein of choice. Eating soy foods will forever be a topic of controversy and one I am not interested in engaging in for this book. But in following the science, controversy, and conflicting evidence on the safety of soy foods, my personal opinion and what we do in my house is this.

We eat soy foods.

Not too much.

We use soy milk in certain things, almond milk in others.

We eat tofu and tempeh but not every week.

We eat steamed, salted edamame, sometimes

We vary our diets like we vary our sexual positions—always trying new things that we've never tried before. Sometimes they're great, and sometimes, shit gets embarrassing.

What about those smoothie places or juice bars?

If it's a true juice bar where they juice fresh fruits and vegetables in front of you, serve shots of wheat grass and the place smells like celery and patchouli, the menu is probably pretty healthy. If you see things like a homemade wild rice burger served on a sprouted grain bun with alfalfa sprouts and heirloom tomatoes, call me and tell me where you are so I can join you. Consider yourself lucky if you have one or more earthy and health conscientious cafés in your city.

What you don't want is a smoothie loaded with milk, added sugar or a mysterious scoop of something powdered followed by squirt of orange juice that comes from a hose attached to the counter where vodka once flowed. Ask to see a nutrient profile of what you're ordering; check how many grams of sugar it contains. Do you remember how many you can have? If not, go back to chapter eight and read it again.

Do the work to find the places you can go and order delicious food you like and that will keep you skinny and healthy. Then the next time you're on the go, you won't have to wonder where to go or what to eat. You'll have those staple places, and good convince meals already figured out. It's worth the initial effort.

As you acclimate to more healthy-ish foods,

hopefully you'll find yourself wanting higher and higher quality ingredients in everything you eat. Perhaps in the future, instead of getting a protein shake, you'll opt for a place that uses fresh blended fruit, spinach, flakes of coconut and a splash of fresh carrot juice. Now *that* sounds divine!

I have to eat on the go all the time. I need options for fast and healthy foods, especially breakfast.

Actually, this is a rather easy problem to tackle. It begins first with a change in mindset that you need to eat meals—or breakfast for some. If someone says you eat like a bird, take it as a compliment, a sign that you have achieved your goals of eating healthy on the go and not too much.

If you insist on the old way of thinking, that you need three meals and two snacks every day, then get out your blue igloo cooler and a whole lot of Tupperware and set aside all of Sunday to map out your battle plan for the week. If you can do this, you are better than I—much respect. Now you will have everything you need for the week packed with you—this is an amazing dedicated feat.

If you are not willing or able to tackle the

aforementioned Sunday prep routine, then follow me down the wellness continuum to a lesser rung of healthy because we are just not there yet or never will be. Let's first salute the dedicated individuals with enough willpower to prep all their food ahead of time. Seriously, jelly as to how they can do it right? Now, let's get fucking real with ourselves and admit that the rest of us might never get there. In this case, quick and healthy day might look like this:

Banana and coffee

Snack food bar

Cranberry walnut salad (eating out)

Handful of peanuts

Pizza

Collapse in bed, hope for a less stressful day tomorrow.

To turn the above day one notch in the direction of healthier on the continuum, maybe it looks something like this.

Banana, coffee, and hardboiled egg (In the car)

Cashews and two oranges (Brought from home)

Cranberry walnut salad (eating out)

Nut crackers and Hummus (brought from home)

Pizza (hubs and kids)

In this scenario you might actually be full from the day and have the willpower to say no to more than one slice of pizza. Cheers, you've made good progress!

Now, get over the idea that you are going to make a healthy dinner for you and everyone else every night—I don't know anyone who can. Worry about yourself until you get all this shit figured out, get *your* weight under control first. Model for them.

To turn the above day one notch healthier on the continuum, maybe it would look something like this:

Breakfast smoothie: grapes, orange, pear, spinach, banana and soy milk. (Or whatever, use ingredients you like). Put half your smoothie in a mason jar and take it with you in a small cooler or insulated bag.

Mid-morning snack: the rest of your breakfast smoothie

Lunch: Very Veggie Sandwich (see recipe)

Snack: Almonds and dried papaya (Yes, you can

have dried fruit. As long as you don't pig out on a whole ton of other carbs through your day, you can have these things. Keep it under control here; dried fruit is very energy dense, so keep it to a handful. If you can't do that then you can't have it.)

Dinner: Let's say you had good intentions but lack of willpower won the fight here and you ate a huge entrée out for dinner with your family. So what! You've had a pretty good run, tried your best, did better than before. Weight loss takes time. It *should* take time if you're going to permanently change your habits. Keep up the good work. Enjoy your night out and have a glass of Cabernet for me.

How much water do I really need to drink? Do other beverages like coffee count?

The boring answer is to drink half your body's weight in ounces of water each day. So if you weigh 140 pounds, your body would need about 70 ounces each day.

In my world, all liquids count toward this daily goal except alcohol. If you pulverize fruit in the Vitamix until it runs from a spoon, it's liquid. Does it contain water? Yes, it's mostly water. Fruits and vegetables are 90 percent water. For fucks sake, why wouldn't you count it?

Coffee is a mild diuretic. But, I don't drink one cup of coffee and piss out one cup of water. The water loss from coffee is not significant if you don't go nuts with it. Coffee and tea both count toward your daily liquids goal. But don't be stupid now and drink a pot of coffee to hit your goal—that would not count.

One or two cups of black coffee each day is plenty, don't ya think? If you feel like you need more then take a closer look at why you think you need it. If it's energy you desire, perhaps getting your ass to the gym at three in the afternoon should be your main concern, because above anything else you could do, exercise will increase your energy levels without a doubt. Cutting out all the crap out of your diet and juicing one day a week will increase your energy levels too.

Let's get to the real question here: "*Will drinking more water help me to lose weight?*" In order for your body to turn fat back into glucose and use it for energy, it needs water and oxygen to be present. So yes, water is important. Oxygen is important. *But* drinking more water than you need won't make you lose weight any faster. It might make you feel fuller longer; cold water might even burn a few more calories for you. If you drink too much around meal times it might also might make you bloated.

Will more water than what your body needs translate into substantial weight loss and really make a difference? No likely. Get in what you need, drink when you're thirsty. Don't be a dummy, of course water is good for you, but it's not going to work like phentermine.

What type of exercise will help me lose weight the quickest?

Like water, oxygen must be present for your body to turn fat back into glucose and use it for fuel. So if you're huffing and puffing during your workout and can't catch your breath, not enough oxygen is present for lipolysis (the conversion of fat back into glucose) to happen.

When your body is not able to use its fat stores to keep your legs going around on the spin bike, it switches mechanisms and burns only available sugar instead (glycogen stored in your muscles and liver.) If you insist on working out at a high heart rate in the absence of oxygen long enough, when your glycogen stores are depleted you will "hit the wall" or literally have no more fuel to keep moving. When this happens or even when someone gets relatively close to "hitting the wall" which for some people doesn't take much, the after effects can be miserable and include vomiting, headache, prolonged lack of energy and extreme fatigue until your body can build back up its glycogen stores again. If you feel like shit after your workouts for a prolonged period of time, this is probably what's happening.

Does it make sense to work out to feel better but the very thing that is supposed to make you feel better actually makes you feel like shit? If you feel like shit after your workouts, (I don't mean muscle fatigue or weakness because you haven't eaten, that is to be expected) you're doing it wrong.

There is a place for high-intensity workouts, interval training and burning the most calories you can on the treadmill by working harder and harder (the cardio zone, as it's posted on most exercise equipment) and you can do those activities; they will help with weight loss, usually. Your body will need to refuel so when oxygen and water are present again, it'll burn body fat to give you fuel.

But remember what I said about exercise—she's a touchy little bitch. Sometimes you can work at the highest intensity you possibly can, and still not burn fat because it can't happen until after your workouts when oxygen is present in abundance like when you're sleeping, if you get enough sleep. And sometimes that conversion of fat to glucose never happens because you ate like shit again and your gains are offset by the Oreos you had to eat because you were so low and depleted from your nutso workout you couldn't resist them.

I was chatting with a friend of mine a few years back and he mentioned that he had cut 30 pounds of body fat in three months as he was getting ready for a body building show.

He set his alarm clock to get up in the middle of the night to eat chicken so that any possibility of catabolic muscle wasting was eliminated. In other words—he ate so much protein and only protein, so that he was ensured not to gain any body fat and at the same time not lose any muscle mass. Sounds fun, don't it? His breath stunk; halitosis, a side effect from a high protein diet when all that animal flesh rots in your gut and its fumes seep back out past your lips.

Anyways, I asked him what he did to prevent muscle wasting and burn fat in regards to exercise. He said, "I walk. Every day, before breakfast. That's it."

From my own experience losing weight and from working with hundreds of bodies through the years, the best exercise to burn body fat is... drum roll please...

Walking.

Not power walking, not jogging, not running. Walking like a normal human walks when listening to music and whistling along happily in the sun. Why is walking the golden ticket? Because when you walk, generally, you take in a lot of oxygen, and assuming you're hydrated, you now have a magic combination to burn body fat (the fat burning zone it's called on the exercise equipment).

One more thing, and this is important. When you start your walk, your body uses its sugar stores as fuel to keep you going. But as time goes by, your body realizes *shit, I don't know how long she's going to be doing this, I'd better conserve my quick sugar stores in case I need them, in case a little kid runs out in the street after a ball and I need to sprint to save him. I can only use quick sugar for that.* So then your body says, *I guess I'd better switch over to burning those fat stores I've been hoarding in case she's going to be doing this a while. And God knows we've got plenty of fat stores to keep her walking to Anchorage.*

This is when the magic happens.

20 minutes into your walk, with water and oxygen, and the fat burning epiphany—your stubborn fat cells are finally giving up their cache. This means, that if you were working with me and your goal was weight loss and you

understood what I've just explained to you, then you would not be resistant to the notion that your "walk" doesn't start until after you've already been walking for 20 minutes. When you walk, if you want to burn fat and see results, you need to walk for 60 minutes. Which actually means you have to walk for 80 minutes. You get me?

If you don't have 80 minutes to walk and try to convince me that you read somewhere to walk 10 minutes at a time and that all those minutes can add up to 80 over the course of the day, I'd ask if you'd been listening *at all* to what I've just explained. Nothing happens after 10 minutes of walking; so what, you've burned off 40 calories, the equivalent of a sick of gum? No deal. If you are truly serious about getting rid of body fat, you'll not tinker around. Recognize that this one thing is a SURE BET for burning body fat. 80 minutes, non-negotiable.

But don't go longer than 80 minutes. If you do, that bitch in the control room gets an alert that you might be trying to trick her again, and she'll pull back the dial on your fat burning capabilities. She'll keep it all in storage where it belongs to save your life in the event there's a coming famine.

What is the best kind of alcohol to drink if I'm trying to lose weight?

We covered this in the last chapter and the answer is, the stuff with the least number of calories, but it's worth re-visiting this question here with a different perspective.

For a period of many years, I was under the impression that alcohol was bad—very bad and that it was the reason I was not losing that last five pounds. Of course I would think this; that information has been stuffed down my throat for twenty years. So begrudgingly, I forced myself, I mean *forced* myself to not have any more than one glass of wine, one or two days a week.

That might seem like a reasonable amount and something to aspire to, but for me, it was giving up a lifestyle of having one, sometimes two, glasses of wine each night with my husband. A time we look forward to more than any other in the day. Our wine ritual comes with feelings of de-stressing and giddy friendship which has produced countless memories of pure bliss with a little fuzzy buzz facilitated by a delicious vining fruit. The experience, the feeling, the time, the winding down, wasn't something I wanted to give up. But I did. I stuck to my self-imposed prohibition for better part of a one summer.

Here's the good part, where I tell you not only did I lose five pounds but I lost 10 pounds by giving up alcohol.

Nope.

Didn't lose a single fucking pound. Not one.

Speculate all you want as to why I didn't lose weight. But I can assure you I have done many experiments on myself and only changed this one factor, my diet and routine stayed the same.

I really don't care why I didn't lose the weight. The more important lesson for me is that I can drink as much wine as I want and for reasons I can only speculate, it does not affect my weight loss or cause me to gain weight.

I wished someone had pointed this out to me before I spent that entire summer dry and grumpy in a boat at the lake. But instead, what had been constantly forced inside my ear drums was that alcohol was bad and that it would make me gain weight and prevent me from losing it. Now this could be true for many people, but it's not true *for me*.

But, I can't drink beer in the same way I drink wine. If I was to have one or two beers each night instead of wine, I'd jiggle a whole lot more in my bikini. My experience here is only with wine—red wine. Not white wine, not beer. The point here is, evaluate carefully what works for you and what doesn't, then you will have the answer to your question.

What about pesticides on produce—is it necessary to wash them with a special soap?

Non-organic produce contains pesticides, period. The actual number of pesticides one piece of fruit generally contains varies as much as the number of sexual partners people have in their lifetime—sometimes one, sometimes 27. If you're concerned, buying organic pretty much ensures no pesticides have been used.

Each year, watch dog groups come out with a list of the "dirty dozen" which usually looks like this: strawberries, apples, nectarines, peaches, celery, grapes, cherries, spinach, tomatoes, sweet bell peppers, cherry tomatoes, and cucumbers. These are the lucky varieties that have proven to contain more pesticides than their sibling counterparts. Depressing isn't it?

We could talk here about all the damage pesticides can do to pregnant mothers, children, your reproductive system, our pets, our soil, our water and just about every other fucking living and non-living thing on the planet *but*

223

volumes have been written, armies have been built, on every side of every issue—including this one. I shalt not repeat all their work which I cannot duplicate as effectively.

If you want to read more about the pesticides that may or may not be causing you cancer and poisoning your water, I've put some resources for this in the recommendations section. Happy reading.

Here's what you need to know. Can you wash the pesticides off? Yes, some. But, in a peach, for example, the residue gets into its skin. You can never wash or cut it all off. So how do you minimize your exposure? Buy organic. When you can't, wash your produce in a solution of 10 percent distilled white vinegar, 90 percent water. When you're pressed for time and just need to rinse that thing under water, do it. I've been known to scrub an apple with Dawn dish soap in my hands ten seconds before I sprint out the door. Does Dawn dish soap work? I don't know, but it makes me feel better than when I just wash things with water or scrub them with my shirt while I'm driving.

What can I order at a restaurant that's still good but won't make me gain weight?

Simple. Water. Bahahaha!

The real answer is that the answer lies within the pages of this book that preceded this page. If you don't know what to order by now from reading chapters 1–14, then go back and try again.

Or you could try ordering an appetizer or sides instead of an entrée. I will often put a few sides together instead of ordering a full meal. Don't order more than you can say "no" to; don't even try to split the entrée in two parts, packing one half for later. You know you'll eat it when you get home anyway. In my house, if that half entrée is still there in the morning, it's lucky to be alive. That's if it makes it to the fridge and I didn't forget it on the table at the restaurant where all the other leftovers go to die. Which is probably the best thing that could have happened to it since it didn't have a chance at my place anyway.

If you think you'll split it and save half for later, you might be tempted to order something especially unhealthy. Perhaps rationalize why eating a smaller portion means that you can order something a little naughtier. At this point you might as well eat it all at once, have another drink and call it your cheat day—go to bed, get heart burn, fart or belch all night then vow to do better tomorrow.

What should I do if I have back pain?

Every time someone asks me a question, I think to myself, "*Am I qualified to answer this?*" No matter the topic, my answer to myself is always "*Nope.*" There is always someone more qualified than I am to be answering pretty much anything. I share *what I think I know* from my bank of some useful and some useless knowledge. If you can take any small thing away that might be helpful, great.

1. Lose weight if you have weight to lose.

2. Start moving your body in ways that feel good.

3. Stop sitting.

4. Do whatever you have to do, quit your job, get a standing desk, get a treadmill desk, pursue a new career that keeps you on your feet and moving but do not sit all day! Walking all day would be better for your back than sitting. If you have to sit for long periods, make every effort to get up every hour and move around and stretch.

5. Do yoga. Gentle yoga. Don't go sweat your ass off in yoga and expect your back to feel better. That kind of yoga is great for the backs that can take it and have worked their way up to that level. Go to beginner's yoga, prenatal yoga, get an at-home restorative yoga video. It

would be much wiser for you to lose any weight you have to lose, and stretch, before pounding your ass on the treadmill or lifting weights. Be kind to your. body.

6. Get help. Go to a massage therapist that knows what they're doing. Better yet, go to a physical therapist that knows what they're doing.

7. If all else fails, go to someone who knows about low or upper backs or wherever your area of concern is. You wouldn't go to a podiatrist to get a boob job would you? No. So don't go to just anyone for your back. Go to the guy or gal who does backs and only backs, all day, every day, and most importantly, *trust them!* They are the ones who know what they are doing. Good luck to you.

What can I do about hormone imbalance?

If you suspect you are imbalanced, take it seriously and get some help. See your doctor. If that does not satisfy your questions, see a different doctor. Go to a compounding pharmacy that deals with bio-identical hormones and speak with someone who knows about hormonal imbalance and what to do about it.

Ask about natural progesterone therapy. Ask if they can point you in the right direction of a doctor who deals with bio-identical hormones regularly. It is my experience working with women and weight loss that if they are going through some major hormonal changes, it can completely change the game. They can do everything right, everything they had been doing before and get very different results. Get some professional help to get things hormonally right—this is so important.

Chapter 16

"TO LOSE WEIGHT AND KEEP IT OFF FOREVER,
YOU HAVE TO FIND NEW STAPLE FOODS THAT
YOU LOVE JUST AS MUCH AS THE OLD ONES."

Find new staple foods.

Do you think skinny people ask themselves *"What can I eat this week that will keep me skinny?"* Yes! Of course they do. Until they don't have to anymore; until they've figured it out; until they are eating foods that keep them skinny without ever having to think about it. Get into the place where your natural go-to choices, your inborn desires, are for foods that are foolproof for your long term weight loss success. To lose weight and keep it off forever, you have to find new staple foods that you love just as much as the old ones.

Replacing your old unhealthy go-tos by filling in the holes with healthy foods you like just as much will take some time and effort. You'll need an open mind, a willingness to try new foods, and time to experiment cooking with them. If you are stubborn and won't try things you haven't heard of, or you have a preconceived negative notion about a certain food, then you're pretty much too stubborn to change. Go ahead then and stay eating the same stuff you've always eaten and get the same results you've always gotten.

Permanent changes will never happen quickly. Change works best when it goes almost unnoticed. So that once you have become the new you, going back to the old you will be just as difficult as it was becoming the new you.

If I cooked for you, came into your house each night, prepared you a flavor-filled colorful dish with leftovers you'd dream about, you'd be broke—but you'd get skinny. Best of all, you wouldn't complain or miss your old crappy foods that were keeping you from your ideal weight.

When things taste good and satisfy our cravings we don't give two hoots what's in them. Hot dogs. You know... spleens and snouts. They're a bad choice, we know it, we still do it (not me).

You will have to learn how to eat and cook differently than you have before if you want to see results.

You can do it. I did it. I was raised on a diet that is very different than the one I have now. Had I kept the diet of my early childhood, I'd likely be overweight, depressed, have colon cancer and my arteries caked with plaque. This was a typical dinner menu in my house when I was a growing up:

Monday:	Spaghetti with venison hamburger.
Tuesday:	Venison tacos.
Wed:	Steak or venison hamburgers and baked potatoes.
Thursday:	MustGo. Everything left in the fridge *must go* into the pot. MustGo.
Friday:	Dinner out. Usually a buffet I now call "The Royal Trough."
Saturday:	"Shit on a shingle" as my Dad would call it. Venison hamburger and gravy over toast.
Sunday:	Fresh fish and homemade French fries.

There were variations of this, but generally, each meal consisted of venison meat until it ran out, coupled with something white and pale yellow. But basically meat and potatoes. I have fond memories of eating like this. I remember loving it; we ate very well and pretty much everything was home cooked.

My folks had no reason to think those were poor choices and certainly not all of them were. The tacos did come with lettuce and tomatoes—which I never ate. What my folks knew at the time is that they were serving us healthy, home-cooked meals, high in protein, minimally processed, with mostly whole foods. I grew up on a home-cooked American diet of meat and potatoes.

Dad told me that when I was a little kid I would say, "More meat, more meat," and that I finished my plate joyfully. I do remember a time of eating meat and having no qualms about it. Of course I was not taken to a slaughter house to see what actually happened, nor was I privy to the chopping of chicken heads at the farm just outside of town. I was never informed that the slab of meat at Easter dinner was Wilbur—it was just meat. I assumed only heathens on the other side of the world were cruel enough to eat pigs and stuff an apple in their mouth. I was confused and surprised when I realized those heathens were me.

I wasn't quite a teenager when I learned all about

what I was really eating and how it got to my dinner plate. It was then I no longer wanted to contribute. When people would ask me what I wanted to be when I grew up, I would answer Marine Biologist. Secretly, I would say to myself *vegetarian.* I fantasized about being a vegetarian (and a mermaid) like other people fantasize about being doctors or lawyers. I wanted to be one of those gutsy people who stuck up for animals and had figured out how not to eat them.

I was not able to make the switch until many years later. A few key things happened that pushed me toward the mostly plant diet I enjoy today.

1. I learned that what I considered a healthy diet of meat and potatoes was probably killing me—clogging my arteries, keeping me fat, messing with my hormones.

2. I found out there were individuals, sometimes whole families, out there somewhere that didn't eat animals—they had learned how to survive on meatless meals. I had absolutely no idea who they were, what they ate or where to buy this special food let alone try and cook it for myself—but if they could figure it out, so could I.

3. I gained the confidence to eat a *mostly* plant-based diet without support or encouragement. More

importantly, I found the strength to block out negative comments about my new plant-eating choices.

4. I had enough money to buy groceries and was old enough to cook for myself.

5. I got sick and thought I was going to die and knew I needed to make the leap from meat-eater to plant eater. I wrote about it *AFFAIRYTALE.* Below is an excerpt:

God—I know it's been a while—and I'm really sorry but I wasn't sure if you were real or not and I didn't want to insult you by praying only when I needed something.

...I need your help.

I know I've been bad—really bad, but this hangover will not go away and it's been five days. I feel like I might die, something's wrong, I feel my life's energy draining out of me.

If you let me live I promise to never, ever eat meat again. I'll stay healthy, and take care of myself, and devote my life to a good cause. Please let me live, and I'll keep my promise OK?

Love—C.J.

And that—is how I became a vegetarian.

Turns out it wasn't a five-day hangover but some

rare pneumonia. I lived anyways and never ate meat again.
Surely my genius boyfriend would see the folly in eating
animals.

I made that promise 14 years ago and have kept it since. I made the switch literally overnight, and I do not recommend doing it that way, but I was long overdue for making that final commitment to a mostly plant diet. I had been wanting to fully commit for years but felt like such an outsider for even thinking about it.

I had exactly zero friends or acquaintances that were vegetarians. Most people I encountered scoffed at my preposterous notion that eating plants was healthier than eating animals. There was a lot of eyeball rolling, "You're too sensitive, everyone eats animals, we have to eat animals for protein" type of discouragement. Since I didn't know a single soul who was a plant eater, I had effectively marooned myself from basically my entire world.

I began spending time at the library where I could seek out others like me in the world regardless of geographical boundaries—sort out all the confusion from what I was hearing and start looking for the truth. It turns out that the truth is hard to find.

My meat-eating roots were not easy to dig up and

sever. I suspect whatever your ingrained habits are won't be easy to change either, but that is not an acceptable excuse to not change. If you would eat what I cooked for you and think you would enjoy it, then you have an obligation to do it without me.

A typical dinner menu in my house now for two adults, one teenager and two toddlers looks something like this:

Monday: Veggie burgers on sprouted multi-grain buns topped with shredded carrots, zucchini, beets, avocado and Dijon dressing. Side salad and/or sweet potatoes with broccoli.

Tuesday: Salmon. Steamed broccoli, asparagus and mushrooms, or cauliflower mash.

Wednesday: Oven baked tofu, well done, slightly crispy with roasted vegetables.

Everyone except my hubs complains about this. I make it in spite of them, and will until they stop complaining.

Thursday:	Super Nachos. Tortilla chips, refried beans, tomatoes, green onions, olives, cheese, homemade guacamole and a cooler cold Corona with a lime.
Friday:	Take-out loaded vegetarian pizza.
Every day:	Green tea in the morning. Red wine in the evening.

On a bad week, our menu looks more like this:

Monday:	Appetizers and drinks at girl's night with my terribly obnoxious friends. Cheat night all night.
Tuesday:	Salmon and steamed vegetables, brown rice.
Wednesday:	Nothing. Every person for themselves. Raid the pantry and refrigerator. Cereal, nuts, granola bars, fresh fruit, pasta from a box, frozen pizza, frozen waffles, toast, stale bagels etc.... whatever happens to be in the house and is generally quick and unhealthy.

Yes, I keep unhealthy things in my house. I have three kids, a husband and a full-time career. I'm fucking busy. Until that changes, we accept life with some convenience foods.

Thursday:	Subway in the car on the way to a family hike.
Friday:	Cheese pizza. Pan. Take-out.
Every day:	Green tea in the morning. Red wine in the evening.

Most weeks look like the former, if they weren't, I'd be a blimp and shouldn't be writing this book. We continue to strive for more quality family time and less on-the-go stress time which almost always harbors unhealthy food choices.

Here is what I *wish* my weeks looked like and sometimes they do, however this does not satisfy all the mouths in my house at present time, so I can't always do what I want. Which makes weight loss or weight maintenance difficult. When my kids are gone and there are less taste buds talking over each other, my weeks will look more like this. Ahhh... I dream of this:

Monday:	Homemade sushi and Sapporo.
Tuesday:	Salmon and steamed vegetables

	with garlic cauliflower mash.
Wednesday:	Homemade spring rolls for lunch. Dinner out, whatever I want with my very witty husband. Sex.
Thursday:	Strawberry spinach almond and feta salad with poppy seed dressing.
Friday:	New recipe night. Sex.
Saturday:	Nothing. Boycott Cooking. Cheat day, all day.
Sunday:	Homemade vegetable lentil soup. Sex.
Every day:	Mimosas for breakfast, green tea for lunch and wine at dinner.

A girl can dream, right?

Find new staple foods that you like and can incorporate into your life permanently. Try a new meal once a week. There are recipes in the back of the book. Be brave, experiment, and remember, it's only kinky the first time.

Chapter 17

A NEW WAY OF THINKING

It's OK to feel a little hungry.

It's deeply ingrained in our biology for us to be continually searching for the next meal. When we find it, we are programmed to gorge ourselves, packing in as many calories as possible.

It seems to me that our innate Homo sapien instinct constantly reminds us that we don't know where or when our next meal is going to be; so eat as much as possible as often as you can. This incredibly useful internal drive to pillage for food is one of many reasons our species is not extinct. We have effectively populated and dominated the planet, swallowing up its resources, simultaneously decimating countless other species who were competing for the same resources in the process. Mission accomplished. We are alive, procreating and fat, while 99.9 percent of all other species that have ever existed are extinct.

The time of hunters, gatherers and opportunistic clans has passed, but it may be a long while, if ever, before our biology trusts the bounty of twenty first century supermarket.

In the meantime, overcome the urge to binge and pilfer when you don't really need the calories to survive and are not even hungry anyway; just bored. Ask yourself, *"When has there been a time I haven't had access to a Goliath number of calories?"* The answer to this question for me in is always... *"Fucking never."*

I now recognize that I am not in a situation of feast or famine, so I can say to myself, *"Listen bitch, if you really want that in an hour, you can just go and get it!"* Then tell yourself over and over until it becomes seared on your brain like a brand, *"It's OK to feel a little hungry."* Create your own affirmations, mantras or mottos that work for you. I'd love to hear them. Tweet them to me @CJEnglishAuthor.

If you want to lose weight permanently and not succumb to the affluent diseases of the Western world (cancer, diabetes, and coronary artery disease), you must figure out how to evolve. We can't wait for a billion more years to pass, hoping our biology can catch up and tell us to stop eating so much and stop eating so many animals.

If we as a species—well, some of us—can overcome the primordial drive to seed our genes far and wide instead of settling on just one mate, we can overcome the biological urge to eat too many calories and be tempted to eat too many animals.

In the Western world, food is everywhere all the time. There is no shortage. I would happily forfeit the variety, access, and quantity of food that is available to me if it were to be shared with the 800 million people who are starving and the 30,000 children dying of starvation around the globe every day. I hope to see and be a part of changing this horrific disparity in my lifetime.

But as long as we have access to an unbelievable number of calories within 10 minutes of our doorstep—dollar menus on every small-town main street in urban America—we'll need to consciously overcome the desire to eat more than we need.

We can do it.

Start by:

Recognizing when you are overeating.

Recognize when you're eating and not even hungry.

Understanding why you do these things.

Only then, when you recognize you're doing it and know why, can you figure out how to change your thinking and thus change your behavior.

...

I suggest journaling every morsel that goes into your mouth while you are trying to lose weight or eat healthier. Write down *what*, roughly *how much*, the *time*, and *what were you thinking and doing*.

Just the act of having to write down what you ate will be a deterrent for eating unhealthy. Take it one step further and post what you ate on the refrigerator for the whole house to see or turn it into your personal trainer or wellness coach each week for a grilling.

Accountability is key.

If you put your money down for it, your time, make a public declaration or have to be accountable for your actions to someone you respect, you'll be more likely to make changes, want to please, and succeed.

After each baby I've had, I've posted a sticky note on the wall in the bathroom above the scale. On the top of the sticky note, I've written my goal weight 115–120 pounds, then hung up a pair of booty shorts close by to look at every day and be reminded. Each week, a few times, I would weigh myself, write the date and my weight on the sticky note and not care who sees it. Although doing this has always been a little scary and vulnerable, I recognize that's only because I don't want to fail and now I've just declared my goals. And once I've declared my goals, I expect myself, and they expect me to follow through. And I have. Every time. I've gone from 170 pounds to 120 pounds in five months after my babies arrived. How did I do it? I've just told you everything I know. Almost.

So go tell someone your goals. Get vulnerable. Stick a post-it on the wall in the bathroom above the scale with your goal weight on the top of it and a pair of booty shorts next to it. Let your husband see and encourage you. If he laughs at you or doubts you or is unsupportive in your efforts to be healthier, tell him to go suck his own dick, then find a good divorce lawyer. Surround yourself with people who take care of themselves and support you in your journey to take care of you.

...

Read.

Lots of books with lots of confusing opinions that require you to think for yourself and figure out what is the truth for you. If you actively search, you will eventually find the answers you seek. But you must think critically along the way. Don't believe everything you read or hear no matter the source.

...

"You may have noticed that you sometimes feel more full about 20 minutes after you stop eating than you did while you were still eating. This is because it takes the stretch receptors in your stomach about 20 minutes to tell your brain (via the hormone cholecystokinin) how full you really are. If you eat until you experience yourself to be 100 percent full, you actually go about 20 percent over capacity with every meal. And if you do that regularly, your stomach will stretch a little bit each time to accommodate the extra food. Then you have to eat more next time to get the same feeling of fullness." (Robbins 2007)

Try thinking about overeating in a different way. How about this: fill your stomach half with food, one fourth with water, and leave the other fourth empty. Wouldn't that feel better than food migrating back up your esophagus and filling your mouth with little bits of throw up because you ate too much?

...

I use this affirmation often:

I like being skinny more than I like [fill in the sinful food here.]

I like being skinny more than I like bread sticks.

I like being skinny more than I like ice cream.

I like being skinny more than I like pasta.

I like sex more than I like to overeat.

Re-train your brain to make better choices using affirmations or statements of motivation that are meaningful and work for you.

I've encountered many women who just won't stop thinking or talking about food. For fuck's sake, isn't there anything else in life besides pasta and cheese? If you need this affirmation, and I've found some of my clients have, then here it is... *stop thinking about food!*

Tell yourself to focus on other things. Eat and be done. Find other enjoyable hobbies in your life besides being a food troll. Chances are when you think about what you might find in the fridge or pantry, it's not because you're hungry, it's because you're bored.

Never eat out of boredom.

If you are a boredom eater, get out your list of things that make you happy.

...

Weight loss happens when you change the way you think about *how* and *what* you eat. The best weight-loss program is an education and not really a program at all.

So, the answer to the question
"WTF am I supposed to eat?" is easy.
For me it's plants—*mostly* plants.
I drink wine and eat plants.

Recipes

There is no shortage of recipes, I know this. The foodies and chefs of the world have far superior concoctions than mine. But I've enjoyed throwing together creations while drinking wine in my kitchen over the years. These are the ones that don't suck and work for me and my family.

Beware: I like to dump shit in without a measuring tool. I've tried to be good and meticulous and include serving sizes but I just can't. Not like we follow serving sizes anyway. If I told you, you could only have 1/4 a cup of cereal, would you really only eat that much anyway? Bahahaha! Of course not, neither would I. I need food I can eat the house down in. For me, most of these recipes fall into that category.

I also like to buy as much already prepared as I can. For example, I don't have time to make spaghetti sauce or sweet chili sauce or sweet and sour. For fuck's sake, I buy it. But I look at the ingredients; I make sure there's no extra shit or sugar in there.

I recognize there are endless variations to each recipe that follows, but since I can't follow directions for any of those, these are my versions of what was once something else.

APPS FOR DINNER

Tomato Basil Bruschetta

When the rest of the family wants spaghetti—meaning noodles with canned sauce—I will often make this bruschetta to pile over a small helping of pasta or spiral-cut zucchini instead.

Bruschetta is generally served with baguettes or some sort of toasted white bread. When eating it this way, I prefer two slices of high fiber, nutrient-loaded bread like spelt or Ezekiel. I cut them into eight small squares, toast them in the toaster, and then drown them in bruschetta. Keep it healthy by making the bruschetta the main focus, not the bread.

Ingredients

4 slices high fiber, nutrient dense bread of choice
Recommended: Sprouted grain, or Ezekiel

2 teaspoons olive oil

1 can basil and oregano diced tomatoes, drained

1 tablespoon dried basil or one handful if using fresh

2–3 minced garlic cloves

2 teaspoons balsamic vinegar

Feta (optional, to taste)

Instructions

Sauté drained tomatoes, minced garlic, and basil in olive oil about 15 minutes or until thoroughly heated. Take off the heat, drain excess liquid then stir in the vinegar. While bruschetta is cooking, toast the bread.

Spray the bread lightly with cooking oil on both sides. Place under the broiler 2–3 minutes on each side or until you've reached desired crispness. This way, it will be crispy outside and soft inside. To save time, throw it in the toaster and call it good. Cut each piece into 4 squares. Top with bruschetta, sprinkle with feta (optional) and serve with red wine.

Sweet and Sour Tofu Skewers

Ingredients

1 red bell pepper

1 yellow zucchini

1 package whole mushrooms

1 small red onion

1/2 cup fresh pineapple chunks

Extra firm fresh tofu (not silken)

Prepare Tofu

Rinse tofu. Slice into two or three slabs. Place a clean dish cloth on the bottom of a baking pan and the tofu on top. Put another clean dish cloth on top of the tofu. Put a stack of heavy books on top of the tofu to press the water out of it. Leave it sit while you prepare everything else. You want as much water out of it as possible so it will absorb the marinade and get crispy on the outside.

Marinade

I use a store bought sweet and sour sauce to save time, but you can make your own marinade if you like or skip the marinade all together and season with sea salt, pepper, or red pepper flakes. Or use your favorite barbecue sauce, sriracha, sweet chili, basically whatever flavor you like you can marinade them in.

Combine tofu, vegetables and pineapple in marinade, leave it sit while you cut the vegetables.

Prepare Vegetables

Cut bell pepper, red onion, zucchini, mushrooms and pineapple into bite-size pieces.

Assemble

Alternate vegetables, pineapple and tofu on skewers. Cook for 30 minutes at 400°F on a lightly sprayed baking sheet or on the grill. Tofu will be soft in the center and crispy outside. Serve with red wine.

Roasted Red Pepper Hummus

Traditional hummus calls for tahini and olive oil but you don't need it to make good tasting hummus, just use the bean water instead. The extra fat calories keep me fuller longer and don't affect my weight or my cholesterol, so I prefer to keep them in.

Ingredients

1 can garbanzo beans (chickpeas)

1 tablespoon cumin

1 cup roasted red bell pepper
Recommended: Jarred is much easier

2 tablespoons tahini

2 tablespoons olive oil

Squeeze of lemon juice

Instructions

In your blender, add drained beans (save the water), cumin, tahini, olive oil and roasted peppers. Blend until desired consistency. Add remaining water slowly if necessary. Serve with nut crackers or raw veggies.

Hummus Deviled Eggs

If the eggs are really fresh, congratulations, and keep buying them, but they will suck for hard boiling. Old eggs are best for peeling after hard boiling. The fresher the eggs, the more difficult it will be to peel them without completely destroying them. You can also try adding 2 tablespoons white vinegar into the cooking water. Either or both of these methods work for me in addition to cooling them very, very quickly after they are removed from the heat. I run them under cold water then put them in the refrigerator to cool asap.

Ingredients

Hard boiled eggs

Hummus

Recommended: see **Roasted Red Pepper Hummus**

One regular size tub of hummus or the recipe above will fill a dozen halved eggs.

Instructions

To hard boil the eggs, place them in a pot and cover with water an inch above the single layer of eggs. Bring to a rapid boil then let stand for 20 minutes. Drain the hot water and replace it with cold water. Let them sit in the fridge for another 10 minutes before peeling. Cut the eggs in half and discard the yolk, replacing it with a dollop of hummus. Or mix the hummus with the yolk. Unless I'm replacing the yolk with only hummus for a different flavor, I prefer to keep the yolk. I always eat the yolk when I eat eggs.

Spring Rolls

There is definitely a learning curve when trying to roll spring rolls, but when you get it right, you'll never again get it wrong. They are SO freaking delicious and healthy and will keep you skinny, so they're worth it. It took me about 10 rolls over two separate meals to get a tight, desirable roll.

This recipe will make 4 spring rolls.

Ingredients

2 Carrots

1/2 Cucumber

1/2 Avocado

4 Lettuce leaves

4 Spring roll wrappers

Sweet Thai chili sauce

Preparation

Slice carrots and cucumbers into really thin strips. I prefer to julienne them; I've used a cheese grater and a mandolin, both work. Don't even think about hand-slicing them unless you want to slice your own hand off, and even then, the taste will not be the same with large chunks of carrot or cucumber.

Wait to slice the avocado until just before you put it in the spring roll.

Assembly

Lay the rice paper on a clean, dry, non-textured surface. I have used the bare granite on my counter, a cutting board and a glass serving tray, all work well. Drizzle about 2 teaspoons of water on the rice paper and use your hand to wet it thoroughly on both sides. Don't wet it too much or it will tear. Keep in mind while you arrange your vegetables that the water will soak into the rice paper and soften it, so don't drown it right away; it'll get softer in a few minutes as you assemble its guts.

Place a palm size leaf of lettuce on the 1/3 portion of rice paper that is closest to you. Inside the lettuce leaf, evenly layer julienne carrots and cucumbers, then slice and place avocado on top or on the side but still in the leaf. Fold the lettuce around the vegetables as much as possible so the carrots and cucumber don't poke through the rice paper. DO NOT OVERFILL or you'll rip it for sure.

Once you have your filling in place, pull the rice paper edge closest to you over the filling sticking it to the other side just in front of the filling. It won't' be tight at this point. Fold in the sides, then pull it all toward you so it gets tight—be careful. Then fold in the sides, pull it in toward you so it's tight and repeat until finished. Use water on your finger to seal any loose edges.

Keep it moist if you're saving it for later, and don't cut it in half until you're ready to eat it to prevent the avocado from turning brown.

Serve with sweet Thai chili sauce.

BREAKFAST ALL DAY

Almond Milk

Don't expect to make almond milk for the first time and not get messy if you're using a flour sack like I do to expel the milk from the pulp. It's messy. If you like fresh almond milk (nothing beats it) and make it often, get yourself a Big Fat Nut Milk Sack from BlankIt! Concepts to make things easier.

Ingredients

1 cup raw unsalted almonds

3 cups water

Nut milk bag, fine mesh strainer or a clean flour sack

Teaspoon of vanilla (optional)

Teaspoon of agave (optional)

Glass storage jar

A really good blender

Instructions

Let almonds soak in water overnight for at least 12 hours. Rinse and discard soaking water. Mix almonds and water in the blender on high for at least 2 minutes. Strain the milk into a glass container via nut milk bag or by pouring over a flour sack and twisting to expel the milk. Discard dry pulp or use for another recipe like crackers—of which I have yet to master so you won't find that here.

Almond Milk Chia with Bananas and Walnuts

Ingredients

2 tablespoons chia seeds

1 cup almond milk

1 teaspoon vanilla

1 teaspoon agave

1 banana

Handful of crushed walnuts

Instructions

I like it when the consistency of this concoction is like tapioca pudding. For that to happen, the seeds need to soak overnight. I have eaten them after they've soaked for two hours and it works just fine, but I prefer a thicker texture. Soak the chia seeds in almond milk with vanilla and agave for at least two hours or overnight. I use a mason jar so I can shake it up in the morning. Add sliced banana and a handful of crushed walnuts just before eating, spoon right out of the mason jar.

2-Minute Oatmeal with Blueberries and Slivered Almonds

If you hate oatmeal because you've only had it served to you in globs of mush with zero texture and flavor, I'm truly sorry you've been improperly fed all these years. Cooked differently, oatmeal doesn't have to be an unidentifiable bland pig slop. Give it the ol' college try one more time for and for God's sake, don't ever cook it in water.

Ingredients

Whole old-fashioned oats (instant oats = mush)

Unsweetened, plain soymilk or nut milk
Recommended: see Almond Milk recipe

Cinnamon

Handful of blueberries

Small handful slivered almonds

Stevia or agave or a little of both

Instructions

This can be made in the microwave or on the stovetop in the same way. Use as much oatmeal as you like, use enough soymilk to cover the oatmeal but not so that it looks like a bowl of cereal. Add cinnamon to taste.

Cook in the microwave 2 minutes then stir it. Do not cook the shit out of this or it will not have any texture. If done properly, the oats will still look like oats when it's done cooking. Microwave about 4 minutes total for a good serving. On the stove top, simmer for about 5 minutes. Most of the liquid will be absorbed but not all. It will be a little chewy, not gooey. Add in frozen or fresh blueberries—bananas and walnuts work well, too.

Add in slivered almonds or other nuts, and use a packet of stevia or a tablespoon of agave to sweeten.

Spinach and Feta Omelet with Chunky Tomato Sauce

Ingredients

3 eggs (local, cage-free)

1 handful fresh spinach

2 teaspoons tomato and basil feta

Spaghetti sauce

Instructions

Use your best non-stick pan or lightly spray a pan with oil. Make an omelet as you regularly would. Beat the eggs, no milk needed, and pour them into the pan. Work the uncooked egg through, around, and under until both sides are fully cooked.

Pack spinach tightly in your hand; tear it into small pieces as you place it over half of the omelet. Sprinkle spinach with feta and close it up. Flip and cook on low heat until it's piping hot inside. Top with traditional spaghetti sauce.

Almond Milk Quinoa

To keep the birds and insects from eating it, quinoa developed a bitter coating of saponins. These natural deterrents make it nearly unpalatable. Most quinoa is pre-washed and free of this bitter taste but look at the packaging to be sure. If it is not pre-washed, be sure to wash it. All you have to do is rinse a few times in a colander.

Ingredients

1/2 cup quinoa

1/4 cup almond milk
Recommended: see Almond Milk recipe

1 teaspoon vanilla

1 teaspoon cinnamon

Stevia or Splenda to taste

Instructions

Cook pre-washed quinoa the night before for a quick breakfast in the morning. Prepare at a 1:2 ratio quinoa to water or as directed on the package. Add almond milk, vanilla and cinnamon to cooked quinoa. Heat thoroughly. Add stevia or agave if desired or fresh fruit just before eating.

MOSTLY PLANTS FOR DINNER

Caramelized Onion and Butternut Squash Casserole

The caramelized onions in this recipe are delicious and easy to make, but they do take some time. Start them first, and they will be sweet by the time you're done chopping vegetables.

Ingredients

1 large yellow onion

1 cup frozen corn

1 red bell pepper

1 yellow bell pepper

2 cups veggie stock

1 cup quinoa

1 large butternut squash

1 package sliced portabella mushrooms

1 tablespoon cumin

1 tablespoon cinnamon

1 tablespoon oregano

1 package feta (optional)

1 small package cherry tomatoes

Olive oil

4 cloves garlic minced or pressed

Instructions

Slice the yellow onion—it does not need to be diced or cut into small pieces, just shoestrings. Sauté the onion in a drizzle of olive oil over low-medium heat. Cover and stir frequently until the onions are soft, brown and have a caramelized look.

Preheat oven to 350°F.

Boil 1 cup quinoa in 2 cups veggie stock until liquid is absorbed. About 15 minutes. Set aside.

Cube the butternut squash*, chop the peppers, mushrooms and tomatoes into bite size pieces, add the garlic and toss together in a large baking dish. Drizzle with olive oil and add cumin, cinnamon and oregano. Mix together thoroughly.

---

* Cutting butternut squash is a bitch. Do not attempt if it's just been plucked from the garden or market aisle. Poke holes in skin, microwave it for at least three minutes, then peel, scoop and cube.

In a separate bowl, mix together cooked quinoa, frozen corn, feta and caramelized onion.

Add the quinoa mixture to the vegetables mixing thoroughly.

Cover with foil and bake 30–35 minutes until veggies are tender.

Perfectly Pan-Seared Salmon

Ingredients

Salmon† fresh center cuts, skin on

Fish or meat spice rub ‡

2 tablespoons coconut oil

Instructions

Clean your fresh cuts so the flesh is free from any rogue scales. Rub the cuts with a very liberal amount of spice rub. If you don't put enough rub on your fillets, they will not get a crusty top.

Melt coconut oil in a large pan on medium heat. When oil is hot, place salmon fillets rub side down. Let them cook until when you look at the sides of the fillets they are halfway done. More importantly, when they un-stick themselves, they're ready to be flipped. If you try to

---

† Don't use this recipe with frozen or frozen-thawed salmon or with salmon that does not have the skin on. Only fresh cuts with the skin on will work for this recipe. Don't worry; it won't go on your plate with the skin. But you want it on when you cook it

‡ Try to find something that does not have any type of salt in the few ingredients. You'll want to use as much rub as the fish will hold to get a crusty top.

move them and they stick to the pan, they are not done. Wait until the rub unsticks itself to turn them over.

Flip and cook the fillets skin side down for another 3–4 minutes or until they are cooked through. DO NOT OVERCOOK or they will be rubbery and chewy and suck.

This is important, so don't skip it. When the fillets are done, wrap them individually in tin foil, and let them sit on the counter for 10 minutes. This "rest" will seal in the natural juices and keep them from getting dry.

Before serving, gently remove the skin. Serve with garlic cauliflower mash.

If you're wondering what kind of salmon to buy that is sustainable, join the club. As I write this, farmed salmon is not ecologically ethical and wild Alaskan salmon is well-managed at the moment. But that could change. To keep a vegetarian diet with a small amount of fish, eggs or dairy requires that you buy those products from sustainable, ecologically friendly sources. If you're going to eat fish, eggs or any type of dairy product, do so responsibly and not in moderation, only in very small amounts for you and for the planet.

Garlic Cauliflower Mash

Ingredients

1 head cauliflower

3 cloves garlic

1 tablespoon vegan cream cheese

Unsweetened, plain almond milk

Instructions

Steam cauliflower and garlic cloves in a steamer basket until the cauliflower is tender. Transfer cauliflower and garlic to a high powered blender, add vegan cream cheese and blend. Add only enough almond milk (in tablespoon increments) to make it creamy, and be careful not to water it down. Work the mix with a spatula or spoon rather than adding more almond milk for a more potato-like texture.

Cowboy Pizza with Guac and Blue Corn Chips

Beans instead of meat, beans instead of meat, *beans instead of meat!* The days of pepperoni pizza are over. Meat lover's pizza is possibly the most heart-unhealthy food on the planet.

Ingredients

1/2 cup frozen sweet corn

1 small jar of pizza sauce

1 can black beans

1 large tomato diced

3 green onions diced

1 extra-large pre-made pizza crust or 2 medium size (personal preference)

Leaf lettuce

2 teaspoons cumin

2 avocados

1 lime

2 teaspoons garlic powder

Organic blue corn chips

Instructions

Preheat oven according to pizza crust package. Mix together drained, rinsed, black beans, corn, diced tomato, diced green onions and cumin. Spread pizza sauce on crust and top with the bean mix. Bake according to the package directions. When pizza is done, top with homemade guacamole, chopped leaf lettuce and crushed corn chips. Eat with a fork

Super Easy Guacamole

Mash 2 avocados in a serving bowl with a fork. Squeeze in the juice of one lime and garlic powder. Add hot sauce or a spoon full of salsa if desired. Stir until stir until desired consistency.

Fully Loaded Bean Tostadas

Beans instead of meat, beans instead of meat, *beans instead of meat!*

Ingredients

1 can fat-free refried beans

Tostada shells

Optional Toppings

Pick and choose what you like or use them all. If serving guests or kids, put all the topping in individual ramekins and let them make their own.

Diced green or red onions

Diced tomatoes

Black olives

Green chilies

Jalapeños

Sweet corn

Cilantro

Salsa

Homemade guacamole

Chopped lettuce

Instructions

Preheat oven to 350°F. Spread refried beans over tostadas. Place on baking sheet. Cook with your favorite toppings. Bake for 7–10 minutes, and add additional toppings when done.

Lentil Taco Filling

You will never miss the meat in tacos after having these. Lentils and beans are great substitutes for beef in almost any recipe. If you are cutting out wheat or flour products to get serious about losing weight, serve the taco filling over a plate of chopped lettuce.

Ingredients

1 small yellow onion, minced

1 tablespoon chili powder

2 cloves minced garlic

2 teaspoons cumin

1 cup red lentils

1 teaspoon Italian seasoning

2 cups and 2 tablespoons veggie stock

Taco shells

Instructions

Add your favorite taco toppings. Sauté onions and garlic in 2 tablespoons veggie stock over medium heat until soft (about 5 minutes). Add chili powder, cumin and

Italian seasoning and lentils. Mix well, then add 2 cups veggie stock. Simmer, covered about 20 minutes or until liquid is absorbed. Serve like tacos, with your favorite fixings, tomatoes, salsa or hot sauce, guacamole and chopped romaine.

Soup-Dish

I get a lot of requests for casserole, hot dish or soup recipes. This one is the best of all worlds. You can have it as soup on Monday night for dinner, then voila, hot dish for lunch on Tuesday.

Ingredients

8 cups vegetable stock

1 cup fresh chopped parsley

1 cup minced onion

1/2 cup lentils

2 cups trimmed, halved fresh Brussels sprouts

1 can drained kidney beans

6 cloves minced garlic

2 cups whole grain pasta shells[§]

1 tablespoon dried basil

[§] Pasta is optional. If you use pasta, have it for dinner as soup then let it sit overnight, the pasta will soak up most of the liquid and make this a perfect hot dish consistency for lunch tomorrow.

1 tablespoon dried oregano

2 teaspoons red pepper flakes

Croutons (optional)

Instructions

Bring the veggie stock to a boil. Add lentils, garlic, onion, beans, parsley, Brussels sprouts, basil and oregano. Turn the heat down, cover and simmer about 30 minutes until lentils and Brussels sprouts are almost tender. Then add pasta, and simmer another 7–11 minutes until the pasta is cooked al dente. Top with croutons if desired.

Spinach and Pesto Quiche

Ever wonder if your grocery store eggs are actually fresh or not? Here's how you can tell. When you crack an egg into the pan, the yolk will be a nice, rounded mound and the white will stay close, raised and taut to the center yolk. If the white is watery and spreads out everywhere with lots of edges, it's old. Find fresh, local cage-free eggs if you're going to eat them. The taste is worth the extra effort.

Ingredients

2 packages frozen thawed, drained chopped spinach

5 eggs

1/4 cup plain, unsweetened almond milk

1 package dry pesto mix

1 cup shredded organic mozzarella cheese

1 jar chunky spaghetti sauce

Instructions

Preheat oven to 350°F. In a large mixing bowl, mix together, spinach, eggs, almond milk, cheese and pesto packet. Pour into a lightly sprayed pie pan. Bake 30 minutes or until eggs are fully done. Top quiche with hot, chunky spaghetti sauce.

Tempeh and Veggie Chimichangas

Tempeh is fermented soybeans. It has a great "meaty" texture. If you've never tried it, this is a great starter recipe. I use tempeh in dishes that would traditionally have used chicken like fajitas. The chimichanga filling is great over a plate of chopped lettuce instead of wraps.

Ingredients

1 small yellow grated zucchini

1 cup diced tempeh

1/2 cup minced yellow onion

6 cloves minced garlic

1/4 teaspoon cinnamon

2 teaspoons cumin

1 tablespoon chili powder

1 teaspoon Italian seasoning

Veggie stock

1 tablespoon balsamic vinegar

Large whole grain wraps (the thinner the better)

Preheat the oven to 400°F.

Instructions

Sauté onion and garlic in small amount of veggie stock and balsamic vinegar until soft, add tempeh (already cooked), grated zucchini and spices. Mix together thoroughly and heat until piping hot.

Spoon the mixture into the wraps and roll like a burrito, folding in the sides. Place the wraps on a lightly sprayed cookie sheet and spritz the outside of the wrap with an oil spray. Bake 10–15 minutes on each side or until golden brown and crispy.

Serve with your favorite condiments. Try salsa or guacamole.

SMOOTHIE JUNKIE

Pineapple Caribbean Smoothie

Ingredients

1/4 cup frozen pineapple

1/4 cup frozen strawberries

1/4 cup frozen mangos

1 tablespoon unsweetened coconut flakes

1 cup coconut water

Handful of spinach or kale

Instructions

Blend. Drink. Go for a walk. Get skinny.

I always put spinach or kale in my smoothies in addition to a greens powder. Yes, it turns them green, but so what, they don't taste green.

Green Smoothie

There are hundreds of green smoothie renditions, and I have tried enough to turn my blood green and morph into a leprechaun. This, or something like it, is my favorite.

If you come to my house and I serve you a green smoothie for dinner instead of an actual dinner, then a glass of wine for dessert, don't be surprised—you wouldn't be the first. It's just how I roll.

Ingredients

1 cup plain soy milk

1 pear

1 banana

1 small bunch red seedless grapes

1 orange

2 cups kale leaves**

Handful ice cubes

** I don't love kale. I prefer spinach, but this trick has made it much better for me. Tear the kale leaves off the center stalk and use only those. The center stalk and veins are what give it a bitter taste when eaten raw.

Instructions

Wash the fruit and kale, core the pear, and toss everything into the blender with soy milk.

This smoothie will get thicker the longer it sets. I recommend drinking half for breakfast and then taking it with you in a glass jar. Have the rest for your mid-morning snack.

Peanut Butter and Chocolate Banana Smoothie

Ingredients

1 cup plain, unsweetened soymilk

1 tablespoon unsweetened cocoa baking powder

1 tablespoon peanut butter

1 banana

2 tablespoons agave

Ice cubes

Instructions

Get outcha' blender! Blend the hell out of it. Serve in a wine glass.

Sinful Chocolate Smoothie

Sometimes I just crave calories or something sweet or something sinful. So, I indulge. This desert smoothie does the trick to satisfy any of those. Buyer beware: it's very high in fat calories.

Ingredients

1/2 cup coconut milk

1 tablespoon unsweetened cocoa powder

1 tablespoon natural creamy peanut butter

2 tablespoons agave

Instructions

Blend all ingredients until creamy. Serve over ice. Sip and be in heaven.

Walnut and Date Smoothie

Ingredients

1/4 cup walnuts

1 banana

2 dried dates, pitted

1 cup rice or nut milk

Handful of ice

Instructions

Blend. Take with you on your way out the door.

OTHER STUFF YOU MIGHT LIKE

Very Veggie Sandwich

Don't skip this recipe or the beets in it. I hate beets, but in this sandwich, they are a must-keep. This is the one recipe to try that you'd never guess tasted so good. I had other veggie sandwich recipes in this chapter but they weren't worthy next to this granddaddy.

Ingredients

1 zucchini

1 carrot

1 beet

Handful of spinach

Handful of sprouts

1 avocado

1 tomato

1 tablespoon tahini

2 slices of a hearty bread, lightly toasted

Recommended: I like to use Spelt bread or Ezekiel for this.

Instructions

Over your cheese grater, grate a small handful of zucchini, carrot and beet. Use 1/4 of the avocado and a thin slice or two of tomato. On lightly toast bread, spread tahini on both slices. Canola mayo works well too, as does hummus.

Layer first with sprouts and spinach then tomato, avocado, beets, carrots and zucchini. I stand on the counter and squish this thing down with all I've got, then slice it and hopes that half of it stays in between the slices as I eat it. But just in case, always bring a fork.

Stewed Apple

Cooked fruit is bursting with antioxidants and is a superb choice to get your digestive fires going in the morning or to "break-the-fast" after a bout of juice fasting.

Ingredients

1–2 tart apples, cut into small pieces, skin on

1 teaspoon vanilla

Agave to taste

Cinnamon (optional)

Instructions

Place small apple pieces into boiling water. Simmer for 10 minutes. Drain. Mix in vanilla and agave nectar to taste. Add cinnamon if desired.

Chocolate Mousse and Fresh Berries

This is the time to get over your fear of tofu. It's a great alternative to dairy in many recipes. For this recipe, use silken tofu, cut the box open, rinse it off and toss it in the blender. It's that easy.

Ingredients

1 box silken tofu firm

2 tablespoons unsweetened cocoa baking powder

1 ripe banana

2–3 tablespoons agave nectar

1 teaspoon vanilla

Soy milk and optional soy whipped cream

Optional tablespoon of instant coffee for Coca Mocha Mousse. 1–2 baskets desired fresh berries

Instructions

In your blender or food processor, mix tofu, cocoa powder, banana, agave, vanilla and splash of soy milk. It should be a thick, pudding-like texture. Add additional soy milk or additional agave for desired sweetness. Top with fresh raspberries or strawberries or use it for dipping berries into. Try topping it with soy whip!

Nut Butter Banana

Ingredients

1 banana

1 tablespoon almond butter, cashew butter, sun butter or peanut butter

1 tablespoon ground flax seeds

Instructions

Slice banana lengthwise. Spread nut butter over each side, then sprinkle with ground flax seeds. Place the halves back together and cut into bite-sized pieces. Store in an air-tight container if you are taking this with you for a mid-day snack.

Nut Cake

No formal recipe is needed for this quick snack, but there was nowhere else to put it. Spread nut butter over a rice cake, top with ground flax or chia seeds if you like, and add sliced bananas.

Ingredients

Any variety rice cake

Any nut butter

Sliced banana

Ground flax seeds or chia seeds optional

Roasted Chickpeas

This is a starter recipe for basic, roasted chick peas. They are delicious like this or in combination with other seasonings. I have tried all sorts of roasted chickpeas and the options are endless: ranch, wasabi, curry, barbecue etc.... I started with these.

Ingredients

1 can chickpeas (garbanzo beans)

Salt or garlic salt

1 tablespoon olive oil

Red pepper flakes or cayenne

Instructions

Wash and rinse chick peas. Blot dry. Transfer to a large bowl, drizzle with olive oil and season with salt and spices or garlic salt. Spread on a baking sheet and bake at 400°F until crispy for about 30 or 40 minutes. Let them cool fully before storing—any moisture at all will make them soggy.

Curried Spicy Nuts

Ingredients

3 tablespoons olive oil

1 cup whole cashews

1 cup whole raw almonds

1 cup pecan halves

1 cup walnuts

Dried spices of curry, cumin and cayenne.

Instructions

Warm olive oil in a large sauce pan—this will make it spread easier across all the nuts. Add spices, about 2 tablespoons each of curry and cumin, then cayenne to preference. Sauté gently for 1 minute to mix all the spices into the oil. Add nuts and coat with spice mixture. Transfer nuts to a baking sheet and bake at 325°F for 15–25 minutes, stirring every 5 minutes.

Cracked Pepper and Parmesan Flax Crackers

Ingredients

1 cup ground flax seeds

2 eggs

1/2 cup fine-grated Parmesan cheese

Sea salt

Cracked black peppercorns or coarse ground black pepper

Instructions

First, preheat your oven to 350°F and spray a baking sheet with nonstick spray—lots of it.

Next, mix ingredients except salt and pepper in a large bowl.

Prepare a surface. I use my counter top and it works great. Another surface may work fine, but you might have to experiment to see what works best. Make sure your rolling surface is thoroughly sprayed with non-stick spray. Spray your rolling pin, too. Do not drizzle oil for a non-stick surface in this recipe, it must be spray oil from a can.

Place your dough ball on the sprayed counter and roll out as thin as you can get it. I like them thinner than any cracker I can get in the store.

Cut into cracker shapes you like (I like them to be not perfectly square or rectangular, I like the jagged edges) use a spatula (sprayed with non-stick spray) to transfer them onto your sprayed baking sheet. Season with salt and cracked pepper.

Bake for 10 minutes then flip and bake for another 3 minutes. To make super crispy crackers, turn off the oven after the first ten minutes, flip them, and then let the crackers sit in the oven for another 20 minutes or more until they are really dry and crunchy.

Agave Pomegranate Lemonade

Ingredients

1/2 cup pomegranate seeds

1 lemon

Agave

Water

Ice

Instructions

Pour pomegranate seeds into a sturdy glass or mason jar then use a muddler, or anything that fits into the jar, to crush the seeds and extract most of the juice. Fill the glass with ice. Squeeze the juice of one lemon over a sieve or fine mesh strainer to prevent the seeds from dropping in. Fill with water, use agave to taste. Shake or stir and enjoy!

"NOTHING WILL BENEFIT HUMAN HEALTH AND INCREASE THE CHANCES FOR SURVIVAL OF LIFE ON EARTH AS MUCH AS THE EVOLUTION TO A VEGETARIAN DIET."

—ALBERT EINSTEIN

(What a freaking genius.)

Afterword

In the late 90's before I was even out of high school, I began to devour diet, nutrition, wellness and weight-loss books—all the well-known, highly publicized ones and dozens of the lesser known often more important ones. I've read journal articles on topics I'm interested in; made a pact with myself to read one scientific article on something related to weight loss each day for a month, for several months. I've followed the controversy over specific foods, GMO's, farming fish, raising bison or grass fed cattle, etc. I read and learn because I want to, because I have a desire to know things and to share things. But finding the truth and deciding what to share has not been easy.

Everything about the food world is convoluted and the more you read the more complex issues become before there is any clarity, if ever. Nutrition science is always changing. There are compelling studies that support every kind of diet, raw food, high-fat, low-carb, plant-based, high-protein, liquid, cabbage soup, carrot soup, juicing, fasting, cleansing, and detoxing every individual organ or organ system. I have asked myself hundreds of times, how do I know who or what to believe? This is what I know; the human tendency is always to be a little biased toward our personal convictions. So how can anything ever be completely truthful? Everything is an interpretation of "facts" with room for error, bias, corruption and the possibility of pushing forth information to further any agenda.

This book is an interpretation of things I've discovered. Not facts themselves, just interpretations and opinions. I support my personal convictions, my opinions, my claims about what is right—for me. Because as the saying goes, if you don't stand for something, you'll fall for anything. I didn't write this book to tell you what to eat or convince you that eating plants is better (OK, maybe I did want to tell you about the plant thing) but more importantly, I wrote this book because I had all this sitting in my head wanting to come out. It was for me. This is my manifesto—a dieter's manifesto. A declaration of what I think I know about eating plants, avoiding eating animals, finding balance in my life, staying skinny, being a good steward while on this planet and figuring out how to navigate this complicated world in general. I wrote this book not to declare some supreme knowledge. I wrote what I wrote because that is how I've interpreted stuff. I wrote this book for me, and if it helps you, great. But what I really want to know is... was it as good for you as it was for me? Bahahaha!

If you enjoyed *WTF am I supposed to eat?* please consider posting a brief honest review on Amazon.

Thank you so much!

C.J.

Recommended Reading

I'm not suggesting you read all of these, some are textbook-like and some are entertaining. My hope is that you find something that is interesting to you and pursue your quest for knowledge about what is healthy and what will work for you and what won't.

In no particular order, except the first one, which everyone should read. Get it on audio book; it's easier to digest that way. And the second one, everyone should read the second one, too.

The China Study by T. Colin Campbell, PhD and Thomas M. Campbell II

Affairytale, a Memoir by C.J. English

Skinny Bitch by Rory Freedman and Kim Barnouin

The Cancer Survivors Guide by Neal D. Barnard. MD and Jennifer K Reilly, RD

8 Weeks to Optimum Health by Andrew Weil, M.D.

Eating Well for Optimum Health by Andrew Weil, MD

Healthy Aging by Andrew Weil, MD

Healthy at 100 by John Robbins

Diet for a New America by John Robbins

The Detox Diet by Elson M. Haas, M.D.

Ultra Metabolism by Mark Hyman, M.D.

The Secret by Rhonda Byrne

The New Optimum Nutrition Bible by Patrick Holford

Harvest for Hope by Jane Goodall

In the Shadow of Man by Jane Goodall

Reason for Hope by Jane Goodall

Prevent and Reverse Heart Disease by Caldwell B. Esselstyn Jr., M.D.

Dr. Dean Ornish's Program for Reversing Heart Disease by Dr. Dean Ornish

The Omnivore's Dilemma by Michael Pollan

In Defense of Food by Michael Pollan

What your Doctor May Not Tell You About Menopause by Dr. John R Lee, M.D. with Virginia Hopkins

The Sexy Years by Suzanne Somers

Breakthrough by Suzanne Somers

Kripalu Yoga by Richard Faulds and the Senior Teachers of Kripalu Center for Yoga and Health

T'ai Chi Chih! Joy Thru Movement by Justin F. Stone

Meditations from The Mat, Daily Reflections on the Path of Yoga by Rolf Gates and Katrina Kenison

Demon Haunted World by Carl Sagan

The Greatest Show on Earth by Richard Dawkins

Crazy Sexy Diet by Kris Carr

Crazy Sexy Juice by Kris Carr

Forks Over Knives by Gene Stone, T. Colin Campbell Jr. Caldwell B. Esselstyn Jr.

Dr. Pitcairn's Natural Health for Dogs and Cats by Richard H. Pitcairn, DVM, PhD, and Susan Hubble Pitcairn

Super Nutrition Gardening, how to grow your own power charged foods by Dr. William S. Peavy and Warren Peary

Safe Foods by Deborah Mitchell

10 Day Green Smoothie Cleanse by JJ Smith

Gorgeously Green by Sophie Uliano

318

Stopping Cancer at the Source by M. Sara Rosenthal, Ph.D.

The World Atlas of Wine by Hugh Johnson and Francis Robinson

The Stark Reality of Stretching by Dr. Steven D Stark

The Oh She Glows Cookbook by Angela Liddon

How to Cook Everything Vegetarian by Mark Bittman

Knife Skills, how to carve/chop/slice/fillet by Marcus Wareing, Shaun Hill, Charlie Trotter, Lyn Hall

The Engine 2 Diet, The Texas firefighter's 28 day save-your-life plan that lowers cholesterol and burns away the pounds by Rip Esselstyn

The Thrive Diet by Brendan Brazier

Monterey Bay Aquarium seafood watch
www.seafoodwatch.org

There are lots more worthy books but these are the ones that come to mind first when recommending something.

Documentaries

Earthlings (2005) Dir. Shaun Monson

Tired, Fat and Nearly Dead (2010) Dir. Joe Cross and Kurt Engfehr

Fast Food Nation (2006) Dir. Richard Linklater

Food Inc. (2008) Dir. Robert Kenner

Forks Over Knives (2011) Dir. Lee Fulkerson

Super Size Me (2004) Dir. Morgan Spurlock

Food Matters (2008) Dir. James Colquhoun and Carlo Ledesma

Hungry for Change (2012) Dir. James Colquhoun, Laurentine Ten Bosch, Carlo Ledesma

King Corn (2007) Dir. Aaron Woolf

The Future of Food (2004) Dir. Deborah Koons Garcia

Acknowledgments

Thank you to Hannah Hutton Clark and Laura Bania who have to fix countless spelling and grammatical errors because I'm a terrible English student but a great story teller. And for letting me know just how much is enough before things get all offensive up in here. It is because of you that I trust and enjoy the writer-editor relationship where I once was down on my luck. Thanks to Mandee at MSPIRE for believing in me from the first day when we had just met over sushi. You've helped give me the courage to put it all out there when I was cold and wet, shivering and looking for a place to hide. Thanks to Cody at Two Hearts Photography for the beautiful cover photo and crazy evening. And to Molly for making me look as good as I possibly could in that insane photo. And to Tyrone at Heritage Homes in Fargo for letting us use that amazing kitchen at the Aspens for the cover shoot. Thanks to my friend whose name rhymes with Schmericka for listening to all my crazy ideas and for knowing that anything you say or do could be the subject of a book at any moment and still being my friend. Nicole, my English teacher friend from somewhere on the other side of the globe of which I'm still not sure where, for taking the time to beta read every word and give invaluable, honest feedback. And to Jeanette, my forever friend; I bet you only said yes to read it early to make sure I didn't use you as subject for a chapter. To Melissa at Rejuv for giving me a homecoming like no other and for believing in me over decades even when eating plants wasn't cool. To all the readers, reviewers and bloggers who helped make *AFFAIRYTALE* a success; I am forever in your debt. I don't know if I would be writing today without your efforts and support. Especially the five that launched it to the top, Allison at Reading Escapade, Flo at Coffee Addict Books, Stephanie at The Belgian Naughty Book Reader, Katy loves romance at Slut Sistas and Kim at Reading in the Red Room. Thanks also to Giovanna at Beauty and the Books, Rachel at Saucy Owl, Dee at Wrapped up in Reading, Martha Sweeney, Vivian at Beaute De Livres, Sher the fabulous book lover, Ellen at The Book Bellas, The Badass Bloggettes, K.K. Allen, Beverly Gardner Tubb, Cassandra at the Bookish Crypt, SueBee, Wenn at Obessessed with Romance, Elizabeth at Crazies R' Us Book Blog, Jenny and Gitte at Totally Booked Blog, Jessica at Jessica's Book Thoughts, Jennifer at Book Bitches, the Page Turning Book Junkie and so many others. You answered my request with an acceptance I was not expecting but will appreciate forever. Mom, thanks for reading it early and giving me your feedback. Sorry I didn't take your advice and take out the part about coconut oil and hand jobs, or the part about not putting a strangers dick in your mouth; or all the overly sexual innuendos you thought were inappropriate; the swearing in general and the self-deprecating tone that undermines just how intelligent you think I might be. I just couldn't bear to delete those things! I love you. And thanks Mom and Dad, for taking the time and effort to cook for us kids and for caring enough to serve us whole foods rather than processed boxes of rice or pasta even if it was animals. I suppose.

To everyone at the lake who insisted on being so much fun every weekend that I couldn't even think about writing; you set back the release date of this book by months and months. I wouldn't have it any other way. To my mother and father-in-law, who despite my foul mouth and embarrassing behavior sometimes, support me anyway. Dani, my teen who saves lives, sleeps too much or not enough, but spends time with me more than I thought possible. Go ahead and buy Starbucks with whipped cream and extra caramel with your own money while you still can. I love you, and the little ones, too. Thanks for being such an amazing and supportive daughter who tolerates my endless stream of sarcasm, listens to all my out-there ideas and still believes that somehow we will become mermaids. Keep believing; dream bigger than you ever thought you could. I wish I had figured that out much sooner. To Jesse for being my #1 fan and supporting me no matter what idea or adventure I have planned next—love you.

My love, sometimes I think about what would have happened if you hadn't adopted a plant-eating lifestyle and had stayed a meat eater. How could I have kissed you? How could we have lived together? We would have had to have two sets of dishes, two sets of pots and pans and two sets of silverware. We might have needed two houses so my clothes didn't smell like cooked meat. Thank God we didn't have to do that, I would have missed you so much and been so lonely I might just have kissed you anyway. You truly are a genius and a gentleman, a more bendable and open-minded person than I. I have learned so much about how to live, love, and keep an open mind to the world because of you. I had no idea life, love, and marriage could be this good. How is it possible that it just keeps getting better? Thank you for your support throughout the writing of this book. Mwah.

Connect with C.J. on social media

www.facebook.com/cjenglishauthor

www.instagram.com/cjenglishauthor

www.twitter.com/cjenglishauthor

www.pinterest.com/cjenglishauthor

Send some love to C.J. via e-mail at
CJEnglishauthor@gmail.com

To inquire about hiring C.J. for a speaking engagement
contact Amanda@MSPIRE.com

References

American Friends of Tel Aviv University. 2013. "Eating a big breakfast fights obesity and disease." *ScienceDaily.* August 5. Accessed September33 2016. https://www.sciencedaily.com/releases/2013/08 /130805131011.htm.

Barnard, Neal D., and Jennifer K. Reilly. 2008. *The Cancer Survivor's Guide: Foods That Help You Fight Back.* Summertown: Healthy Living Publications.

Bingham, SA. 1988. " Meat, starch, and non-starch polysaccharides and bowel cancer." *Am J Clin Nutr* 762-7.

Campbell, T. Colin, and Thomas M. Campbell. 2005. *The China Study.* Dallas: BenBella Books.

Esselstyn, Caldwell B. 2007. *Prevent and Reverse Heart Disease: The Revolutionary, Scientifically Proven, Nutrition-Based Cure.* New York: Avery.

Goodall, Jane, Gary McAvoy, and Gail E. Hudson. 2005. *Harvest for hope : a guide to mindful eating.* New York City: Warner Books.

Haas, Elson M., and Daniella Chance. 2012. *The Detox Diet, Third Edition: The Definitive Guide for Lifelong Vitality with Recipes, Menus, and Detox Plans.* Berkeley: Ten Speed Press.

Holford, Patrick. 2006. *The New Optimum Nutrition Bible*. Berkeley, Calif.: Crossing Press.

Jakubowicz, Daniela, Maayan Barnea, Julio Wainstein, and Oren Froy. 2013. "High Caloric intake at breakfast vs. dinner differentially influences weight loss of overweight and obese women." *Obesity* 2504-2512.

Ornish, Dean. 1996. *Dr. Dean Ornish's Program for Reversing Heart Disease: The Only System Scientifically Proven to Reverse Heart Disease Without Drugs or Surgery*. New York: Ivy Books.

Patisaul, Heather B, and Wendy Jefferson. 2010. "The Pros and Cons of Phytoestrogens." *Frontiers in Neuroendocrinology* 400-419.

Physicians Committee for Responsible Medicine. n.d. "Cancer Resources." *Physicians Committee for Responsible Medicine*. Accessed September 29, 2016. http://www.pcrm.org/health/cancer-resources.

Pollan, Michael. 2006. *The Omnivore's Dilemma: A Natural History of Four Meals*. New York: Penguin Press.

Robbins, John. 2007. *Healthy at 100: The Scientifically Proven Secrets of the World's Healthiest and Longest-Lived Peoples*. New York: Ballantine Books.

Rose, DP, AP Boyar, and EL and Wynder. 1986. "International comparisons of mortality rates for cancer of the breast, ovary, prostate, and colon, and per capita food consumption." *Cancer* 2363-71.

Schwarzbein, Diana, and Nancy Deville. 1999. *The Schwarzbein Principle: The Truth about Losing Weight, Being Healthy and Feeling Younger.* Deerfield Beach: Health Communications.

Walter C. Willet, M.D. 2012. "How Stress Can Make Us Overeat." *Harvard Health Publications.* January. http://www.health.harvard.edu/healthbeat/how-stress-can-make-us-overeat.

Weil, Dr. Andrew. 2012. "Carbohydrate Density: A Better Guide to Weight Loss." *The Huffington Post.* October 12. http://www.huffingtonpost.com/andrew-weil-md/carbohydrates-weight-loss_b_1937312.html.

Excerpt from *AFFAIRYTALE, a MEMOIR*

AFFAIRyTALE

My Love,

You were so worth the wait.

"IF A MAN COMMITS ADULTERY

WITH THE WIFE OF THY NEIGHBOR,

BOTH THE ADULTERER AND THE ADULTERESS

SHALL SURELY BE PUT TO DEATH."

—LEVITICUS 20:10, 538

Prologue

I didn't mind flying, but not like this. I hadn't prepared for this. I wasn't supposed to be taking this long trip alone. Nausea rolled through me in waves.

"Now boarding all passengers on flight twenty-two fifty-six to Kahului. Please have your passes ready at the gate."

I stood up, stretched my legs and got in line at the gate. I was dreading the grueling flight.

The gate attendant scanned my pass. "Thank you, Ms. Summers," she said.

I walked through the narrow jetway, tugging my carry-on stuffed full with bikinis.

It would be the first time I put on a bikini since the surgery. The scars across my stomach and back were still numb and jagged. They still looked fresh. I would stare at someone who had scars like mine. Scars that ran along a spine like a two lane highway, scars that were out of place on a youthful body.

Nightmares about my joints shattering into a million pieces still kept me awake at night. I would crumble brick by brick until I was nothing but a pile of broken rubble.

Normally I wouldn't be scared to travel alone, but on this trip, I feared I would collapse again and not be able to get back up. I would have to crawl on my hands and knees down the narrow aisle, pushing my suitcase in front of me just to get off the plane.

I tried to get comfortable, but my back hurt, my ears rang, and tears wet my eyelashes. I stuffed a pillow between my seat and the window, closed the shade, and squeezed in purple earplugs. I gagged down a Dramamine, but it got stuck, adding to the large lump lodged in my throat already. Loneliness tucked me in with a thin red blanket and offered me its cold shoulder in the place where his should have been. Emotionally exhausted and on the brink of a meltdown, I was a felony disaster.

A few months ago, he'd asked me if I was up for an adventure, and I always was. I loved our adventures, like the time we'd shimmied across that rickety footbridge over the raging Temperance River, or when we had thrown human body-sized logs into a rushing gorge just to see how we might die. The adventures I loved the most were the ones at sunset, like the time we'd laid concealed among the tall grasses looking up at the sky. We watched in awe as one, two, then three bald eagles soared overhead. I adored the many nights we'd slept outside under a million stars, and made love.

We'd made extraordinary love.

We'd hidden when we had to. Those had been the sultriest nights. Locked in his candlelit bedroom where he'd taught me the tango and the rumba, and played his guitar as I lay naked under his cool sateen sheets. I'd been longing to lie between those sheets for nearly a decade.

Now, after all that, the empty seat next to me wasn't my idea of an adventure. It was a heartbreaking reminder of how desperately I needed him in my life, a flashback of how painful it was to live without him. We'd come so far, overcome the impossible, now the grand finale was me, alone.

Maybe I was finally getting what I deserved for what I had done.

The loud speaker crackled, "Ladies and gentlemen, from the flight deck, this is your captain speaking. Our flight time today is seven hours and fifty-one minutes. Looks like clear skies all the way to Maui."

***

U are my wish:)

Chapter 1

Twelve Years Earlier

The pink neon sign glowed *"Psychic"* in the midnight darkness.

I had been driving home after a long shift of serving bar food and beer when I saw it blinking in the window, like a beacon calling for lost souls. Souls like mine, discontent souls looking for answers and comfort within a life of uncertainty and dis-ease. Something urged me to turn around.

The psychic's face was youthful, and her hair bounced with voluminous curls as she walked toward me.

"I don't know why I'm here," I said.

Without another word she led me to a small rectangular table where I sat down, pulled my tip money out of my pocket and laid out twenty crumpled up one dollar bills on the table, her fee for half an hour.

The psychic talked with her hands. "Something is wrong with your car," she said.

I shrugged and shook my head, "I don't think so."

"Yes," she insisted. "Something wrong with your car and you need to get it fixed."

I rolled my eyes. *This is already a waste of my time and twenty bucks.*

I didn't care about my car. I wanted to know about what every nineteen-year-old girl wanted to know about—my love life. "My boyfriend. Is he the one?" I asked.

Without hesitation and with a sense of absolute certainty, she said, "This man you are with is a fine man, and if you want to make it work with this man, you can." She leaned over the table toward me, her eyes commanding my full attention. She continued, "but if you stay with this man, it will be difficult, very difficult." She paused, and then what she revealed next made my heart beat in wild thumps, "the man you are destined to be with is still out there."

It was enchanting—the idea that there might really be one true somebody for everybody. That maybe my somebody was still out there, waiting for me, and that just maybe, she was going to lead me to him.

She reached over the table, wrapped her warm, soft hands around mine, and held them as if she were extracting information from my skin.

"You haven't met him yet, but you will. He has dark skin like yours and dark hair. He is very handsome."

I tried not to show how enthralled I was with her prediction. I didn't want to give any obvious signs that I was buying what she was selling, but involuntarily, an enormous smile grew on my face at the thought of *him*.

She closed her eyes as if to admire him and collect further information from the ether.

With a look of surprise and delight, she continued, "You will know it's him because of his eyes. They are the color of ice. It would be a great love, a rare love, with this man."

Then, as if my body knew something my mind did not, a shiver came over me, and my heart pounded even harder against my chest as she divulged more thrilling information.

"If you choose this rare love," she went on, "it will be the greatest love you have ever known. You are one of the lucky ones."

Every hair on my forearms stood up like I'd been zapped with electricity.

She spoke faster now, information quickly coming to her, "You will have three children with two different men, but this path can change. It has not been decided yet."

Great. Several children with different men? I can't wait to tell my mom.

"If you decide to make it work with the man you are with, it will be hard. Your love will grow cold, and you will become bitter. You will never be truly happy."

Blood pooled in the soft pith of my throat, the way it does when my heart flutters out of rhythm. I didn't want to make the wrong decision. I couldn't dump my new boyfriend because of the prediction of some psychic lady.

What if she's is wrong? What if Levi is the one?

I wanted Levi to be the one. I needed him to be the one. I didn't want to wait anymore. I hated being alone. I liked being loved, and Levi did love me. If he proposed, I would say yes. I would make it work. Like she said, it might be hard, but if anyone could make it work, I could.

Crazy gypsy. What does she know?

The bells on the door jingled as I walked past the neon sign and outside into the night. My mind raced with thoughts of my future, of my here and now, of my car.

My car was parked under a tall, dim streetlight. As I walked up, I took a quick look at all four tires to make sure they weren't flat.

Nope.

I slid into the driver's seat and quickly locked the doors. I fastened my seat belt and wiggled the key into the ignition. After half-expecting it not to start, I was relieved when the engine fired up without a hitch.

Huh. See?

I punched the gas and fled the shady, run-down neighborhood. It was the kind of neighborhood that was eerily silent and dark at night, the kind of neighborhood that allowed an old, white house to become a psychic's studio.

I was heading for the safety of the streetlights when I saw it.

Is that a crack?

It was a crack, one that hadn't been there before, and now, there it was, a lightning bolt that zigged and zagged horizontally across the center of my windshield.

I'll never know if the crack in my windshield was what she had been referring to, but if it were, she was right about that, and a few other things, too.

Although I didn't know it was *him* when it happened, the man with dark hair and eyes like ice showed up in my life only a few months later.

However, I wasn't single, and he was far from being available. In fact, I walked right into his wedding.

***

It was late summer when my older brother Dylan married his high school sweetheart. Lacey was an intelligent blonde beauty, and he was an aspiring bodybuilder with a gigantic laugh that matched his mountainous muscles.

A wildflower garden of yellow sunflowers and lavender hollyhocks stood tall around the well-manicured lawn. Rows of white chairs lined each side of a weathered boardwalk that weaved its way to the altar. Everything that could be was adorned in satin bows and burgundy lilies.

As Dylan kissed his new wife, wedding guests holding small plastic bottles wrapped in silver tulle blew thousands of multicolored bubbles into the air. The shimmering bubbles floated down, landed on our posh attire, and then exploded into a soapy mist. The wedding party, myself included, trotted down the boardwalk and disappeared behind the tinted glass of a polished white limousine.

An entourage of stretch limousines took the wedding party from bar to bar and dance floor to dance floor, with champagne flutes and shots of Grey Goose in between. My limousine shuttled me immediately to the reception for fizzing, tangy punch until some distant relative was kind enough to by an underage girl a drink to celebrate her brother's wedding.

When the bride and groom arrived at the reception they walked through the doors of the Crystal Ballroom where hundreds of well-dressed guests greeted the regal couple with roaring applause. Lacey was stunning in a timeless princess gown entwined on the arm of my brawny brother as she floated effortlessly through the ballroom. They looked and seemed like a perfect match in every way possible.

I wanted that. I wanted to find someone who belonged with me like the stars belonged with the sky. Someone I could get lost in, who would make me forget about reality for a while, who would adore me second to none.

I wanted the fairytale. Perhaps I could have that with Levi. I didn't know. It was still too new to even invite him to my brother's wedding.

A thin partition split the chandelier lit ballroom down the center, and I could hear music coming from the other side. With my burgundy bridesmaids dress bunched up in both hands at my sides I wandered over to check it out. From the hallway the door pulsed with music. It was another wedding, another bride getting her fairytale.

I had to peek inside and see how beautiful and beaming she was on the happiest day of her life. I wanted to see how enamored her groom was by her. I wanted to see the magical way a man looked at his new wife on their wedding day, like she was the only woman on earth.

Just before I was about to intrude something caught my eye. Handwritten in elegant calligraphy and centered inside an ornate baroque frame were two words:

ENGLISH WEDDING

I gripped the oversized door handles, slipped inside, and was greeted by the warm glow of hanging glass. This room was also ultra-posh and filled with its own luxurious amenities, like glittering champagne flowing from two tiered fountains, elegant ice sculptures, and chocolate rivers. The tone was set for an unforgettable night of celebration. The crowd was jubilant and tipsy, and people seemed to move as one organism across the polished wooden floor. Bliss lingered heavy in the air.

It only took a moment for me to spot the bride and groom. He was a dashing gentleman with his arm around the waist of his new wife. They smiled and laughed as they moved through the crowd, exchanging pleasantries and receiving congratulations.

Jealous of their jovial fate and feeling the intrusiveness of my presence on their most beloved day, I slipped out and closed the doors.

Eventually, I would learn that on that inauspicious summer night, nothing was as it'd seemed.

***

*We're still on for
2morrow night, right?
Mwah!*

Chapter 2

Three Years Later

At the top of the stairs of our tiny twin home, an argument of gargantuan proportions ensued. Every muscle in my body wanted to push Levi down the stairs.

We'd met on ladies' night. I had been underage, using a fake ID, and he had been the guy swinging hand over hand from the rafters above the dance floor. Levi was spontaneous and daring. I didn't have to try to have fun with him, he had enough fun for the both of us. He was the perfect escape from loneliness. He showed up with a carefree spirit and lived in the moment, but his recklessness was contagious. Being with Levi had become destructive and addictive.

Looking back, it had been volatile from the beginning. Although it was that very volatility that had made us want to kill each other that had also kept us together. Our personalities clashed, but the clash gave us variety and excitement.

I'd once read couples fight about three things—money, sex, and parenting. In the three years after Dylan had gotten married, Levi and I had become engaged, and we regularly battled over the latter two.

Our first two years together had been great, filled with sex, parties, and enough quality time to meet double my emotional needs. It wasn't until year three when I'd found out I was pregnant that things became complicated.

I was twenty-one when I had Danielle, and I'd quickly realized that our party lifestyle wasn't how I wanted to raise a child. I'd vowed to become the best mom I could, finish college, and do something productive with my life. So that was exactly what I had done. My priorities had changed, so I had changed.

Through college I excelled, checking off one degree then starting another, always sprinting toward another life challenge. I had quickly established a booming career working for myself consulting with private clients and corporations on health and wellness, as well as teaching part time at a local University. I was well spoken, on my way to receiving a master's degree, and employable with a plethora of credentials in health and nutrition. Despite the success, I was hopelessly discontent.

Through the lens of Levi's hazel eyes, all he wanted was for me to be content, for me to slow down, stop bouncing my knees and for once, be happy with what I had in front of me. He was the guy who could stay in a job for two decades with a yearly three percent raise and be satisfied.

I wished I could be that way, I just couldn't. I was a chronically discontent, obsessive compulsive overachiever.

Levi and I were very different. We had conflicting opinions on just about everything that was important to us. We struggled to find balance between our family and our relationship. It didn't seem so uncommon to have a difficult relationship like ours. In fact, it seemed to be fairly normal, like most of the other relationships I'd seen.

We rarely agreed on anything and regularly engaged each other in petty arguments over problems like inequitable household chores or opposing libidos. These arguments became a frequent and toxic cloak over our relationship and smothered our future.

Every sentence began with, "You always," or, "You never," and since no argument was ever fully laid to rest or resolved, snippets of previous arguments were continually reconstituted and poured back into the pot, making a more concentrated poison each time we fought. It was a poison laced with resentment over everything that had ever been said or done that hadn't been resolved. This resentment ate at me from the inside, callousing my heart and turning me into someone I was not.

Resentment killed my spirit in a record quick time. I became a hardened, empty partner lying dead on a cold metal table with a toe tag that read, *"Don't fucking touch me,"* and, *"Don't even dare try to have sex with me."*

We circled each other like bloodthirsty hyenas in a perpetual power struggle. Hating each other over everything that had ever happened, yet nothing was really worth fighting for. The bottom line was that not only were Levi and I not compatible, at some deep biological level we were also lethal to each other.

Violent words spewed off my tongue.

"I hate you."

"I wish you were dead."

"I wish I could fucking kill you."

My mouth was stuck wide open, covering years of ground in just minutes as I unleashed a hellfire of words until words weren't enough. Then, like a feral animal, physical anger forced its way out from inside of me to get its share of the kill. I wailed and kicked and screamed and pushed him down the hallway, lining him up with the stairs. I wanted to hurt him more than I had ever wanted to hurt anyone before. I wondered if I actually could kill him. Was I capable of that? Was that the mental derangement lawyers called temporary insanity? Had I slipped into the state of mind where a woman wanted to lop off her husband's penis?

He stumbled as I tried to launch him down the stairs, but not even a shot of angry adrenaline could give my five foot four inches and one hundred twenty pounds the power to push him more than a few wobbly inches. He easily restrained me. I flailed my arms and legs, trying to jolt free, but my efforts were futile. Levi was thick, not huge like my brother Dylan, but he was lean and muscular. He'd been an athlete in high school and he was still agile and strong.

When he finally let go, the evil inside of me rose up again but it was another failed attempt to overpower him. I conceded. I ran in to our bedroom and locked myself in but not because I was scared of him or what he might do. He would never hurt me. I was frightened by my own psychotic break and the ease at which I could abuse.

I had become the alpha abuser. I was the horrible partner who verbally and physically abused, and I hated myself for it. I hated the person I'd become in our relationship.

That night I cried then slept, then cried. He never knocked on the door to see if I was alright, and I never apologized. I didn't even know what we had been fighting about. Pointless arguments had become a familiar pattern and created a hatred that lingered between us.

After each freak-out, I always regretted my uncouth behavior, but inevitably I would be pushed to my breaking point again and throw more berserk tantrums later. Each one made me a little less whole and a little more crazy.

***

God, it just sucks that
we can't do what we want.
2 stay together tonight.

347

Chapter 3

Dani and I were sitting cross-legged on our lakeside patio, coloring with sidewalk chalk, when I heard Dylan yelling from the end of the dock.

"Come here, quick!" He was looking up at an endless ocean of blue sky.

Dani stumbled as I tugged her plump little hand alongside me. Nanook trotted behind us, tongue flopping and white froth dripping from his black gums. Summertime in Minnesota was brutal for my Siberian husky but a glorious warm vacation for me.

Just as we reached the end of the dock, a red-and-white plane swooped down unusually low, buzzing what seemed like inches from our heads.

I instinctively ducked. "What the—who is that?" I asked Dylan.

He squinted with his hand over his eyes, following the plane through the sky. "Grant," he said.

***

The cabin was nestled into a hillside surrounded by lush Minnesota forest. Our backyard sprawled out into a secluded wetland that morphed ubiquitously into a hundred miles of rolling hills in the Land of Ten Thousand Lakes.

The cabin itself was a time capsule that hadn't changed since 1979, the year I was born. There was carpet in the bathroom, no shower, and curtains hung where doors should have been. The well water tasted like pocket change, and the electricity went out with every summer thunderstorm. Although Mom made sure we had the fanciest cabin on the lake with a lit palm tree, pink plastic flamingos, and a handwritten sign by the toilet that read: "Here in the land of sun and fun, we never flush for #1."

Dylan and I were natural-born lake kids who never missed a weekend. We didn't care that we had to bathe in sixty-degree lake water and sleep in bunk beds that smelled of mold. The cabin was our warm summer reprieve from the icy cold Minnesota winters. Now that we were grown, the cabin was the only place Dylan and I could reunite with our parents before they flew back to their Arizona home each winter.

That night, pale pink and tangerine smudged the Western sky. The sunsets over the cabin were enchanting, each one a unique fingerprint yet each one the same. The wetlands surrounding our evening bonfire seemed to come alive at night. Toads and tree frogs croaked, fireflies blinked across the expanse of the damp marsh, and the resident pack of coyotes bellowed their lonesome howls into the darkness.

Dylan and I were sitting on tree stumps, listening to the crackle and smack of the fire and sipping our sweating Coronas when he asked:

"Where's Levi this weekend?"

I was always ashamed to answer, and my answer was always the same.

349

"Working," I'd say.

Or I'd make up some other lame excuse about how Levi needed to mow the lawn or repaint the kitchen for the sixteenth time.

"What?" Dylan replied, "Tell him to get down here, he's missing out. Work can wait, the summer is way too short to miss a weekend."

The truth was, Levi just wasn't a cabin type of guy. Missing a weekend was his vacation.

"It's too boring there," Levi would say. "What am I supposed to do all weekend? I don't like sitting around all day on the deck or in the boat."

I did. Doing nothing at the lake on the dock, or deck, or in the boat with an apricot brandy slushy were the best parts of lake living, and I wasn't about to cut my time short. It was my escape to solitude. It was the place where, if only for an hour, I could get lost in the woods without anyone caring.

My mom and dad were happy to see their granddaughter and occupy her for hours and hours. Every weekend, Dani and I would pack up our beach stuff and leave Levi behind on the hot pavement of our city home to head for the lake.

As a car approached our cabin its blinding headlights drowned out the color of the flames.

"Who's that?" I asked as a car door slammed shut.

Dylan didn't answer. He never answered—not to me, not to anyone. If he didn't like the question or didn't want to talk, he just simply didn't answer. For no other reason than it was just his way.

When we were kids he was the kind of brother who shot me with a rubber-band gun while I was sleeping and clipped his toenails in my bed. He made me walk ten feet behind him to school and showed me how to stuff my winter coat behind the bushes because "walking to school in a coat is so not cool."

A car door slammed shut and the slap of flip-flops coming toward us grew louder. Dylan stood up to greet the stranger.

"Hey, bud! Glad you could make it."

"Hey, Dylan. Thanks for inviting me."

I was instantly flustered by this man's good looks. He had an All-American smile that was intimidating and distracting.

"This is my sister," Dylan said.

They both looked at me.

I mustered out a clumsy, "hi."

"C.J., this is Grant," Dylan said. "He's the one with the plane from this morning."

"Very impressive," I nodded in Grants' direction.

He was humble and gave a polite, "thanks, nice to meet you."

I went back to doing nothing on my tree stump as they engaged in casual conversation. Except I *was* doing something; I was secretly analyzing this handsome stranger like an undercover agent would analyze her newest assignment. I listened intently as he and Dylan spoke. It seemed like they knew each other but hadn't spoken in long time.

Grant was well spoken, kind mannered and unusually intelligent. Though he also seemed a little distant, perhaps a little lost.

I twirled my engagement ring, alternating it between my middle and pinkie fingers, as I reminded myself: *Ignore him. Stop looking at him. What are you doing? You already committed to Levi, you're taken.*

After thirty minutes I'd gathered that Dylan and Grant had already become good friends, they'd talked on the phone regularly and even planned his stop by our fire tonight.

"Come on, bud. Join us for a few more drinks." Dylan said as Grant finished his beer. "We're going to hit the lake bars after this one. It'll be fun. Come with us."

"No thanks Dylan, I can't tonight but I will sometime soon," He said.

I was secretly excited and terrified to hear that he'd be back and that he was already a close friend of Dylan. *How could I have not known about his super-hot friend before?*

I knew the answer, Dylan was secretive, not a gossip, he'd only tell you what you needed to know in real time. He hadn't been hiding his hot friend, he just never thought to tell me about him.

Then Grant looked at me and nodded. "C.J., nice to meet you. I'm sure I'll see you again soon."

It was in that moment I first saw his eyes. They were nearly transparent, a shade of blue I'd never seen before. They were mesmerizing.

As soon as Grant's headlights disappeared into the dense blackness of the rural road, Dylan leaned forward like he was about to tell a ghost story at summer camp. He set his meaty forearms down on his thick thighs and inched to the edge of his stump.

"It's so terrible," Dylan said, his face twisted in disgust. "Grant's wife cheated on him three months after they were married."

"What? That's terrible. What happened?"

"I don't really know all the details. I haven't seen him in years. All I know is that they were high school sweethearts, and he was with her since he was seventeen."

Who in the hell would cheat on that? I thought.

"I ran in to him a few weeks ago," Dylan said. "I feel so terrible for him. C.J., Grant is the nicest guy. I always knew he had a cabin but I never knew it was on our lake! Can you believe that? He's been on the lake all this time and we never even knew it. It's so great to have another person we can hang out with now."

Our lake wasn't big, not more than a mile across, so it was weird that we never knew he was there, but not impossible. We stayed on our side of the lake, knew our close neighbors but that was all. Knowing someone across the lake was like knowing someone who lives six blocks down.

Dylan reached his thick hand into the cooler and pulled out two more longnecks. "Guess what?" He said, "You're never going to believe this. Grant was the guy who got married on the same day I did. Remember there was a wedding party next door to us in the Crystal Ballroom?"

"Yes, I remember." I said, "I looked in there. That was *him*?"

"Yes. He plays in a band, too. Country music, like us." Dylan was thrilled as he told me about his new friend who we seemed to have so much in common with.

In fact, I'd never seen Dylan like someone so much. He wrenched off the beer tops and handed me a dripping bottle. I flung the ice-cold water back on him but got no response.

"We talked about buying a wakeboarding boat together," Dylan said.

"Really?" I gulped and coughed, immediately feeling panicked that this handsome man was going to be around a lot more. "When? You mean, like, this summer?"

"No. The season is almost over. Now is the best time to buy a boat for next year. C.J., it'll be so fun. We'll be able to do all the things we've never been able to do behind Mom and Dad's boat."

I'd known Grant for thirty minutes, and already I felt like getting married to Levi was the wrong thing to do. Forget about the arguments, everybody argues, if I could be so smitten with another man almost immediately then maybe I was with the wrong person.

It didn't matter how I felt. I'd said yes. We had a child, I could never back out now. Besides, he treated me fine, he wasn't abusive, and he took care of Dani and I. What more did I need?

I soon found out what I needed was someone who I was so enthralled with that the thought of anyone else didn't even exist, which is exactly what happened during the remaining summer. However, it wasn't my soon-to-be-husband who stole my attention.

Surprise appearances from our new friend were becoming more frequent, and my high school crush on my brother's new best friend intensified. I tried to curb my appetite for him. I tried to reason with my mind, but he just kept coming around. Every. Single. Weekend. My fever never had enough time to cool down. Over the course of only a few months, he became like a festering ulcer of guilt and desire.

It wasn't only me who lusted over him. Everyone he met seemed to immediately fall in love with our new single and talented friend.

Dylan had a group of regular friends who frequented our place on the lake, as well as a revolving door of new friends he'd meet and invite over. There were always neighbors around, and my parents had friends and family stop by sporadically too. There was never a shortage of bikini clad bodies lying on the dock or hanging out on the lawn paying bocce ball or throwing a Frisbee.

It didn't take long for Grant to become a part of our regular group. He'd stop by with his new, shiny silver Jet Ski and offer take anyone waterskiing or just take them for a ride. He helped Dani fill up water balloons and instigate a war. We played ladder ball and tossed bean bags and did all the things lake-people do. Just like that, Grant had become a regular fixture with us. No one could believe he'd been right under our noses all those years.

"Who's the new hot guy? Why is he still single?" Our friends and neighbors would ask.

Even my parents doted over him. After Grant brought over his guitar and played music with them, they were instantly enamored with his charm. When he wasn't around they'd ask where he was and why they hadn't met him before and ogle over what a talented musician he was. They sold him vitamins and exchanged phone numbers.

They were right to swoon. He had an enticing charisma that drew you in. After saying not more than a few polite words, he held you captive. Men and women alike seemed to adore him.

Why would a smart, handsome entrepreneur with mysterious eyes and dark hair be single? I often wondered and wasn't the only one.

He was frequently assumed to be either gay, or too damaged from his first marriage to ever settle down again. No one, especially me could believe he wasn't taken.

"He's picky," Dylan would say when someone asked. "He'll never settle."

Grant was irresistible to everyone, except for Levi. They'd met less than a handful of times since Levi was seldom at the lake, but Levi would hear how people talked about Grant. How Grant was a pilot and a musician, a business owner and taught ballroom dance. He actually sounded like a fictitious character when people would list his attributes. I could see how it drove Levi nuts.

When the summer ended, I was surprised at how quickly my schoolgirl crush went with it. Everyone went back to their winter homes and regular lives. During the winter months, we rarely saw each other. Nine months passed without a single glimpse of him. In that time Grant faded in my mind, existing as only an apparition in the long gray winter.

***

Summertime arrived again, and overflowing ponds and streams became home to the returning waterfowl. My chapped winter skin rejoiced in the sun. With the first dose of vitamin D I'd had in nine months, my seasonal winter gloom lifted.

It was a new summer, a new beginning, and just as soon as I settled into my weekend routine, it began: Grant and I were slowly becoming friends, it was as if we'd both missed each other. My spark for him had ignited again. He looked at me, and truly saw me. When his crystalline eyes met mine, everyone else in the world seemed to fall away. My infatuation was back with vengeance.

Our friends and neighbors gathered around the fire to sing and dance in the sand and enjoy the summer libations. There were harmonicas, washboards with plastic spoons, drumsticks on logs, twelve-string guitars, and everyone sang along.

Grant was a jukebox that didn't need a quarter. You could just put in your request and get a personal serenade.

"Grant, play Bon Jovi."

"Grant, play 'Hotel California.'"

"Grant, play Keith Urban."

His brain was a catalog of music he'd collected over years of singing and touring. Playing all genres and every weekend around the bonfire, he wooed us with his encyclopedia of songs. Grant was a modern prodigy, a musical muse. He lured me in with his tenor and then held me captive with his timbre.

The weathered picnic table of my childhood creaked as he shifted his weight, situating his guitar on one knee. I watched him from behind the flames. He was plain and gorgeous— gorgeously plain, in worn-out jeans and an unkempt tousle. His face was bronzed, his voice smooth, and his transparent eyes drew me in closer. I could almost smell his breath and feel the vibration of his words on my skin. He closed his eyes as he sang my request—a love song, of course. Every syllable sent me deeper into a lucid dream, a dream in which I imagined what a life with him might be like.

I floated on the melody, exposing the curves of my neck, secretly inviting him in. When he opened his eyes, they met mine. He looked away, looked back, and then continued my request as if he were singing to my heart alone.

Is he singing to me or just in my general direction?

I analyzed further, examining his body language, where he looked, whom he looked at, and what it all might mean.

Is it possible? Could he be feeling the way I'm feeling? Why does he keep looking at me? Is it a nervous tic or something?

When the fire fizzled out and only the weekend warriors remained we would make our way down to the water and take a midnight ride in the new boat.

Grant and Dylan bought that wakeboarding boat they'd talked about, and stored it right outside my bedroom window.

That summer I found myself in a conundrum worse than any before. I was engaged, tied to Levi with a mooring rope, but I couldn't stop thinking about someone else. All week, I would look forward to the weekend, hoping to get a glimpse of him—the man who just happened to be Dylan's best friend, the man who I'd never seen with a girlfriend because he was so picky, the man who had been cheated on, the man I would never be able to have.

So why not leave Levi? I asked myself dozens of times and the answer was always the same.

I loved Levi. Levi loved me. Things weren't great but they weren't terrible. We had our dark moments, but everyone does. Why would I call off our engagement for a crush? For a man who is way out of my league? No, I would stay with Levi.

This thing that I feel for another man is completely normal, I convinced myself, *a biological desire for the opposite sex, an inborn chemical attraction that would eventually dissipate.*

It didn't, and it seemed that nothing could uproot the seed that had been planted in my subconscious. I had a wanton desire for Grant that kept growing even under the most inhospitable conditions. For reasons I didn't yet understand, I became inextricably bound to him.

***

I will always take care of u
always... sucks that I can't completely
be my loving, caring self around others.

Chapter 4

It was no surprise when Levi turned a shade of jealous green the night I walked away with Grant. Had Levi gone missing with an alluring, charming, multi-talented female—if *they* had wandered out of sight and couldn't be reached—I would have dumped his ass. That's what he should have done to me. Even if Grant had been just a friend, which technically that's all he was—having a male friendship, especially one complicated by my secret emotional affair, was unacceptable and I knew it. I just couldn't help myself.

Check out the *AFFAIRYTALE* book trailer on YouTube

https://youtu.be/zUDhKkyKol0

Or get it here

https://goo.gl/uzabbp